"Brian Wansink is the Sherlock Holmes of food . . .

discovering one reason after another how our food world drives us to eat. We would each do well, the nation would do well, to be mindful of what he recommends."
—Kelly D. Brownell, Ph.D., Director,
Rudd Center for Food Policy and Obesity,
Yale University, and author of *Food Fight*

"Anyone who eats should read this book! Brian Wansink will help you take control of the subtle influences in your environment that can persuade you to overeat."
—Barbara Rolls, Guthrie Chair in Nutrition, Pennsylvania State University, and author of *The Volumetrics Eating Plan*

"A must read for everyone with a serious interest in diet and health."
—Tim Hammonds, Ph.D., President and CEO,
Food Marketing Institute

"Whether or not you're a parent, you owe it to yourself to read Brian Wansink's lively and eye-opening book. You'll never look at your dinner table or your kitchen the same way again."
—James O. Hill, Ph.D., Professor of Pediatrics, University of Colorado Medical School, and author of *The Step Diet Book*

"Enjoyable and filled with fascinating research, *Mindless Eating* explores how our daily food choices contribute to our—and our nation's—increasing girth. Wansink's practical approach reveals that small changes in our daily habits can help reverse this trend."
—Rebecca Reeves, DrPH, RD, President of the American Dietetic Association, and Managing Director, Behavioral Medicine Research Center, Baylor College of Medicine

Mindless Eating

Why We Eat More
Than We Think

Brian Wansink, Ph.D.

BANTAM BOOKS

New York   Toronto   London   Sydney   Auckland

MINDLESS EATING
A Bantam Book / October 2006

Published by Bantam Dell
A Division of Random House, Inc.
New York, New York

Book design by Ellen Cipriano

Bantam Books is a registered trademark of Random House, Inc.,
and the colophon is a trademark of Random House, Inc.

Library of Congress Cataloging-in-Publication Data
Wansink, Brian.
Mindless eating : why we eat more than we think / Brian Wansink.
p.   cm.
Includes index.
ISBN-13: 978-0-553-80434-8
ISBN-10: 0-553-80434-0
1. Compulsive eating. 2. Food habits—Psychological aspects. I. Title.
RC552.C65W36 2006
616.85'260651—dc22   2006047532

Printed in the United States of America
Published simultaneously in Canada

www.bantamdell.com

BVG   10 9 8 7 6 5 4 3 2

To my tireless past, current, and future
co-authors, colleagues, and students,
and to the patient academic journal editors
and insightful reviewers
who make our work better.

Contents

Introduction:
The Science of Snacking

EVERYONE—EVERY SINGLE ONE of us—eats how much we eat largely because of what's around us. We overeat not because of hunger but because of family and friends, packages and plates, names and numbers, labels and lights, colors and candles, shapes and smells, distractions and distances, cupboards and containers. This list is almost as endless as it's invisible.

Invisible?

Most of us are blissfully unaware of what influences how much we eat. This book focuses on dozens of studies involving thousands of people, who—like most of us—believe that how much they eat is mainly determined by how hungry they are, how much they like the food, and what mood they're in. We all think we're too smart to be tricked by packages, lighting, or plates. We might acknowledge that *others* could be tricked, but not us. That is what makes mindless eating so dangerous. We are almost never aware that it is happening to us.

My lab's research has shown that the average person makes well over 200 decisions about food every day.[1] Breakfast or no breakfast? Pop-Tart or bagel? Part of it or all of it? Kitchen or car? Every time we pass a candy dish or open up our desk and see a piece of gum or a PowerBar from 1997 we make a food decision. Yet out of these 200-plus food decisions, most we cannot really explain.

But what if we could? If we knew why we ate the way we do, we could eat a little less, eat a little healthier, and enjoy it a lot more. This is why when it comes to what we eat, lots of people are interested. Getting people to eat healthy foods in the right amounts is of interest to dietitians, calorie counters, and physicians, but also to brand managers, parents, and even governments. It's also of interest to the U.S. Army, *Better Homes and Gardens,* and whoever's making your dinner tonight.

Since founding the Food and Brand Lab in 1997, I have designed and conducted over 250 studies, written over 100 academic articles, and made over 200 research presentations to governments and governors, to top universities and companies, to culinary institutes and research institutes, and I have presented my research results on every continent but Antarctica. Many of the studies in this book have been reported on the front pages of the *Wall Street Journal* and in the *New York Times* and *USA Today.* They have also been reported in the *National Enquirer, Annals of Improbable Research,* and *Uncle John's Bathroom Reader.* They've been featured multiple times on *20/20,* the BBC, and other network TV shows, and they've been bantered about by Rush Limbaugh and berated by Dr. Laura.

I'm on a mindless-eating mission. Still, I'm never sure what to say when someone asks how I first became interested in food, psychology, and marketing. I usually say, "I really liked Vance Packard's 1957 book, *The Hidden Persuaders,* because he tried to show how advertising unconsciously influences us. I think this also happens when we eat, except the hidden persuaders are the way we set up our tables, our kitchens, and our routines."

While that's true, it's not the whole truth.

MY BOYHOOD SUMMERS WERE spent with my brother and cousins on my uncle and aunt's 138-acre farm near Correctionville, Iowa. The highlight of the end of every summer was the day Aunt Grace and Uncle Lester took us to town to see a movie, followed by a stop at a place I remember as the Dairy Freeze.

But in 1968, grain prices were low. When I innocently asked Uncle Lester why we weren't seeing a movie that year, he summarized the state of agricultural economics in seven words, "We would if people ate more corn." To an 8-year-old, this pretty much translated into "If I ever hope to see a movie again, I'd better think of a way to get people to eat more vegetables."

Fast-forward to 1984.

With a newly minted master's degree in communication research, I was working on a consulting project for *Better Homes and Gardens (BH&G)*. One day, the director of editorial research, the late Ray Deaton, showed me four different *BH&G* cover ideas for an issue that was being published in 10 months. All four had the same cover photo and looked identical when I first saw them from four feet away. When I moved closer, I discovered the only thing that differed: the six "cover blurbs," or teaser phrases, on the left side of the cover. Ray asked me to predict which cover would sell the most copies and why. I pointed to one and said, "I think this one will do best because it uses shorter, little phrases." Without blinking, he said, "Your intuition just cost us over a million dollars in newsstand sales." He went on to explain that every month *BH&G* took the best ideas for cover stories, developed four or more sample covers with a different mix of blurbs, and then asked over a thousand nonsubscribers which version they would be most likely to buy off the newsstand. With a circulation base of over 7.2 million readers, they did not use hunches and intuition. They did research so they could predict which magazine a blond, 37-year-old Wisconsin mother of two would pick up, flip through, and buy when standing in the checkout line at Safeway.

I was stunned. I was also hooked. Maybe I could learn to predict what foods people would eat—even if they themselves could not.

Within six months I had applied to a Ph.D. program in Consumer Behavior at Stanford, telling them that I wanted to do research on how to "get people to eat more vegetables." Six eye-opening years later, I was a marketing professor at the Tuck School of Business at Dartmouth College, with a fuzzy dream of starting a food psychology lab.

A "LAB" MAY CONJURE up images of test tubes, bubbling beakers, arcing electricity, and researchers with Einstein hair. Sometimes this is close to the truth, even in food research. Consider the physics of French fries. The Argonne National Laboratory helped McDonald's discover how to speed up the time it took to cook French fries. A team headed by physicist Tuncer Kuzay put sensors inside frozen French fries to best determine how to deal with the steam that was created by melting ice crystals. They then designed special frying baskets that cut 30 to 40 seconds off the frying time for each batch.[2]

In contrast, food psychology labs typically study human behavior, and these labs look like mock living rooms, kitchens, or restaurants. Some might be rigged with one-way mirrors, camouflaged cameras, and tables that have hidden scales under the plates. Others might include a row of cramped three-feet-wide tasting booths where people can taste-test different foods without being distracted. Still others might have small soundproof rooms for in-depth interviews or larger rooms where groups are brought in to answer psychological surveys related to food.

There are dozens of psychology labs that study food either part-time or full-time. They can be found at great universities in the United States, Britain, Canada, the Netherlands, France, Germany, Finland, and elsewhere. They can be found in the U.S. Army. Some of the more secretive ones can even be found in food companies.

Each of these labs uses different methods to study how we eat. But what all the noncommercial labs have in common is that they aim at publishing their findings in the best academic journals they can. Journals like the *Journal of the American Medical Association (JAMA)*; *British Medical Journal (BJM)*; *Obesity Research*; *Journal of the American Dietetic Association*; *International Journal of Obesity*; *Journal of Consumer Research*; *Appetite*; *Journal of Marketing*; *Food Quality and Preference*; or the *Journal of Marketing Research*, to name just a few. Most of the researchers in these labs hope that what they publish will help make people's lives better. Does it? A lot of it is pretty much ignored. But the 10 percent that does make a certifiable difference is the reason many of these researchers will never retire—even when they're no longer being paid.

In this book, I'll refer most often to four labs that have shaped the questions I see as particularly significant.[3]

• **The University of Illinois Hospitality Management Program.** One strength of the HM Program at the University of Illinois in Urbana-Champaign is its research restaurant, the Spice Box. This facility has been used by Jim Painter and myself to study how menus, lighting, music, wine, waitstaff, and dining companions influence how much we eat and how much we enjoy the food. It's open only one to two evenings per week, and it costs less than $25 for an elegant, candlelit, white-tablecloth meal. This is a win-win-win situation. Diners get great meals, students get great experience, and researchers get great studies. The insights discovered there about menu design, food descriptions, food presentation, and ambience are coveted by the food industry, including leading restaurant chains. With dozens of people involved in each research project, many of these results accidentally leaked out to company newsletters and planning meetings months before they were officially published in an academic journal.

• **The Penn State Department of Nutritional Science.** This is the home of Dr. Barbara Rolls' lab, where innovative work with food formulations has shown how variety and caloric density influence how much we eat. If you've read one of the popular weight-loss books *The Volumetrics Weight-Control Plan* or *The Volumetrics Eating Plan,* you are familiar with some of their work.[4] The lab's food buffet has conclusively proven to the food industry that it can design profitable, lower-calorie foods that consumers love to eat.

Dr. Leann Birch's lab, also at Penn State, has done much of the most clever pioneering work on how children eat, showing—among other discoveries—that they're just as susceptible to being fooled by food tricks as adults.

- **The U.S. Army Natick Labs.** As Napoleon famously said, "An army marches on its stomach." Food is a big part of morale in the Armed Forces, as well as a key component of physical readiness and endurance. The strength of the Army Natick Labs is in sensory evaluation, and this lab has employed or hosted about every leading expert in the field. Nearly every day of the year researchers use nine high-tech, computerized taste-testing booths to discover how foods taste differently when they're eaten in the dark, or when they're given bogus expiration dates, or when they're eaten off paper plates instead of olive drab plastic. Led for 40 years by Drs. Herbert Meiselman and Armand Cardello,[5] the experiments in this lab helped the Army learn how foods can be developed, packaged, and served in ways that make soldiers enjoy them more—and eat them all.
- **The Cornell Food and Brand Lab.** This is my own lab, now relocated from the University of Illinois at Urbana-Champaign to Cornell University. Our focus is on the hidden persuaders around us that influence how much we eat—and how much we enjoy it.[6]

One part of the lab is connected to my office and to viewing rooms by two-way mirrors, hidden cameras, and sensors located under dinner plates. In less than three hours we can transform the lab to look like a kitchen, or a dining room, or a living room, or a den with a big screen TV. This lets us examine how the placement of the food on the table, the size of the plates, the type of lighting, or the kind of television show people watch—among dozens of other variables—influence how fast they eat and how much they eat. We bring people into the lab for lunch, dinner, parties, or a snack and we carefully watch and measure what they do under these different conditions.

If a study shows something "works" in the lab, we next test it in "real world" settings. We've gone to Chicago movie theaters, New Hampshire restaurants, Massachusetts summer camps, Iowa grocery stores, Philadelphia bars, Michigan diners, San Francisco homes, and U.S. Army bases, and we have interviewed or surveyed people in nearly all of the contiguous forty-eight states. We're looking to see if the same factors that work in the lab also influence everyday people in everyday situations.

Incidentally, all of these studies are preapproved. Today, each study planned by university researchers must be submitted to that university's Institutional Review Board to ensure it won't harm the participants.[7] Why would someone participate? If they're college students, they usually get extra credit. If they're "real people," they're paid $10–$30, or given free food, movie tickets, and so on. Their identity is always protected—whatever they say and do is anonymous, and any record of their participation is eliminated once we analyze the data.[8]

As I mentioned, many of the larger food companies have in-house labs that typically do taste tests. That is, they pay consumers to try a new food or a reformulated recipe, and to rate whether they like it or not. Although most of these companies are also interested in food psychology, few of them employ the specialists necessary to design subtle experiments and analyze seemingly confusing data. That's why they often come to the academic labs for help or advice.

Some labs, like ours, have a policy of not working directly for food companies. This eliminates conflicts of interest, and enables us to immediately publish our results in scientific journals and to share them with health professionals, science writers, and consumers. But because all labs need money to buy food, pay graduate students, and keep the lights on, this also means we rely on grants and gifts. We've had pieces of projects funded by consumer organizations and by grants from the Illinois attorney general, National Institutes of Health, National Science Foundation, U.S. Department of Agriculture, Council for Agricultural Research, and the National Soybean Research Center. In most years this has worked well and has provided freedom and a sense that good things were happening. In other years, I've had to cover the deficit out of my own pocket. We do the research we think is most urgent and interesting, and *then* we try to find a way to pay for it.

There are dozens of other food labs around the world, and I'll acknowledge their work as it comes up, but most of the research described here is from my own Food and Brand Lab. First, I can provide the sometimes ridiculous "color" of what happened. Second, the studies were planned to be interlocking pieces of a big story about the hidden food persuaders in our lives and how we can make mindless eating work in our favor.

Is This a Diet Book?

To those of us who love food, a diet is pretty much "die" with a "t" on the end. (In fact, "diet" comes from a Latin word which means "a way of life.") I love a great meal. My wife graduated with honors from Le Cordon Bleu culinary school in Paris, and we both passed the first level of certification to become French-certified wine sommeliers. Yet although we end many evenings with a candlelit dinner and a full-bodied glass of wine, I start many mornings with a fast-food breakfast and a full 32-ounce Diet Coke. Reporters often seem puzzled—even semi-disapproving—with my dietary "way of life." I love all food—the sublime, the ridiculous, the refined, and the gross. Like a parent who loves his or her children no matter how different they are, I love the *galette de crabe* at Le Bec-Fin, the Cini-minis at Burger King, and the braised duck tongue at the night market in Taipei.

This book is not about dietary extremism—just the opposite. It's about reengineering your environment so that you can eat what you want without guilt and without gaining weight. It's about reengineering your food life so that it is enjoyable and mind*ful*.

Food is a great pleasure in our life—not something we should compromise. We simply need to shift our surroundings to work *with* our lifestyle instead of *against* it. This book uncovers the hidden persuaders that lead us to overeat and shows us how to eliminate them. On the other hand, if you are running an Army food service, coaxing people to eat in a nursing home, or simply catering to fussy eaters in your home kitchen, the same research can show you how to encourage them to mindlessly eat more of the healthy food that they need.

Traditional diet books focus on what dieticians and health practioners know. This book focuses on what psychologists and marketers know. There are no recipes—only scientifically based findings. Marketers already know some of what you will read, and they use it relentlessly so that you buy their hamburger instead of their competitors'. But this is not an evil conspiracy. Some of the tactics they use are the same ones your grandmother used to make sure you had a great Thanksgiving dinner, and they are ones you can use to make your next dinner party a success.

Traditional diet books lead most people to throw up their hands in frustration and deprivation and to buy another diet book that might promise a less painful way to lose weight. Instead, this book shows you how to remove the cues that cause you to overeat and how to reengineer your kitchen and your habits. You won't be a swimsuit model or a Chippendale dancer next week, but you *will* be back on course and moving in the right direction. You can eat too much without knowing it, but you can also eat less without knowing it.

The best diet is the one you don't know you're on. Let's begin.

The best diet is the one
you don't know you're on.

1

The Mindless Margin

DID YOU EVER EAT the last piece of crusty, dried-out chocolate cake even though it tasted like chocolate-scented cardboard? Ever finish eating a bag of french fries even though they were cold, limp, and soggy? It hurts to answer questions like these.

Why do we overeat food that doesn't even taste good?

We overeat because there are signals and cues around us that tell us to eat. It's simply not in our nature to pause after every bite and contemplate whether we're full. As we eat, we unknowingly—mindlessly—look for signals or cues that we've had enough. For instance, if there's nothing remaining on the table, that's a cue that it's time to stop. If everyone else has left the table, turned off the lights, and we're sitting alone in the dark, that's another cue. For many of us, as long as there are still a few milk-soaked Froot Loops left in the bottom of the cereal bowl, there is still work to be done. It doesn't matter if we're full, and it doesn't matter if we don't even really like Froot Loops. We eat as if it is our mission to finish them.[1]

Stale Popcorn and Frail Willpower

Take movie popcorn, for instance. There is no "right" amount of popcorn to eat during a movie. There are no rules of thumb or FDA guidelines. People eat however much they want depending on how hungry they are and how good it tastes. At least that's what they say.

My graduate students and I think different. We think that the cues around us—like the size of a popcorn bucket—can provide subtle but powerful suggestions about how much one should eat. These cues can short-circuit a person's hunger and taste signals, leading them to eat even if they're not hungry and even if the food doesn't taste very good.

If you were living in Chicago a few years back, you might have been our guest at a suburban theater matinee. If you lined up to see the 1:05 P.M. Saturday showing of Mel Gibson's new action movie, *Payback,* you would have had a surprise waiting for you: a free bucket of popcorn.

Every person who bought a ticket—even though many of them had just eaten lunch—was given a soft drink and either a medium-size bucket of popcorn or a large-size, bigger-than-your-head bucket. They were told that the popcorn and soft drinks were free and that we hoped they would be willing to answer a few concession stand–related questions after the movie.

There was only one catch. This wasn't fresh popcorn. Unknown to the moviegoers and even to my graduate students, this popcorn had been popped five days earlier and stored in sterile conditions until it was stale enough to squeak when it was eaten.

To make sure it was kept separate from the rest of the theater popcorn, it was transported to the theater in bright yellow garbage bags—the color yellow that screams "Biohazard." The popcorn was safe to eat, but it was stale enough one moviegoer said it was like eating Styrofoam packing peanuts. Two others, forgetting they had been given it for free, asked for their money back. During the movie, people would eat a couple bites, put the bucket down, pick it up again a few minutes later and have a couple more bites, put it back down, and continue. It might not have been good enough to eat all at once, but they couldn't leave it alone.

Both popcorn containers—medium and large—had been selected to be big enough that nobody could finish all the popcorn. And each person was given his or her own individual bucket so there would be no sharing.

As soon as the movie ended and the credits began to roll, we asked everyone to take their popcorn with them. We gave them a half-page survey (on bright biohazard-yellow paper) that asked whether they agreed to statements like "I ate too much popcorn," by circling a number from 1 (strongly disagree) to 9 (strongly agree). As they did this, we weighed their remaining popcorn.

When the people who had been given the large buckets handed their leftover popcorn to us, we said, "Some people tonight were given medium-size buckets of popcorn, and others, like yourself, were given these large-size buckets. We have found that the average person who is given a large-size container eats more than if they are given a medium-size

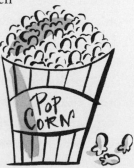

container. Do you think you ate more because you had the large size?" Most disagreed. Many smugly said, "That wouldn't happen to me," "Things like that don't trick me," or "I'm pretty good at knowing when I'm full."

That may be what they believed, but it is not what happened.

Weighing the buckets told us that the big-bucket group ate an average of 173 more calories of popcorn. That is roughly the equivalent of 21 more dips into the bucket. Clearly the quality of food is not what led them to eat. Once these moviegoers started in on their bucket, the taste of the popcorn didn't matter.[2] Even though some of them had just had lunch, people who were given the big buckets ate an average of 53 percent more than those given medium-size buckets. Give them a lot, and they eat a lot.

And this was five-day-old, stale popcorn!

We've run other popcorn studies, and the results were always the same, however we tweaked the details. It didn't matter if our moviegoers were in Pennsylvania, Illinois, or Iowa, and it didn't matter what kind of movie was showing; all of our popcorn studies led to the same conclusion. People eat more when you give them a bigger container. Period. It doesn't matter whether the popcorn is fresh or fourteen days old, or whether they were hungry or full when they sat down for the movie.

Did people eat because they liked the popcorn? No. Did they eat because they were hungry? No. They ate because of all the cues around them—not only the size of the popcorn bucket, but also other factors I'll discuss later, such as the distracting movie, the sound of people eating popcorn around them, and the eating scripts we take to movie theaters with us. All of these were cues that signaled it was okay to keep on eating and eating.

Does this mean we can avoid mindless eating simply by replacing large bowls with smaller bowls? That's one piece of the puzzle, but there are a lot more cues that can be engineered out of our lives. As you will see, these hidden persuaders can even take the form of a tasty description on a menu or a classy name on a wine bottle. Simply *thinking* that a meal will taste good can lead you to eat more. You won't even know it happened.

As Fine as North Dakota Wine

The restaurant is open only 24 nights a year and serves an inclusive prix-fixe theme dinner each night. A nice meal will cost you less than $25, but to get it you will have to phone for reservations and be seated at either 5:30 or 7:00 sharp. Despite these drawbacks, there is often a waiting list.

Welcome to the Spice Box.[3] The Spice Box looks like a restaurant; it sounds like a restaurant; and it smells like a restaurant. To the people eating there, it *is* a restaurant. To the people working there, it's a fine dining lab sponsored by the Department of Food Science and Human Nutrition at the University of Illinois at Urbana-Champaign. The Spice Box is a lab where culinary hopefuls learn whether a new recipe will fly or go down in flames. It's a lab where waitstaff discover whether a new approach will sizzle or fizzle. It's also a lab where consumer psychologists have figured out what makes a person nibble a little or inhale it all.

There is a secret and imaginary line down the middle of

the dining room in the Spice Box. On one Thursday, diners on the left side of the room might be getting a different version of the shrimp coconut jambalaya entrée than those on the right. On the next Thursday, diners on the left side will be given a menu with basic English names for the food, while those on the right will be given a menu with French-sounding names. On the Thursday after that, diners on the left side will hear each entrée described by a waiter, while those on the right will read the same descriptions off the menu. At the end of the meal, sometimes we ask the diners some short survey questions, but other times we carefully weigh how much food our guests have left on their plates. That way we don't have to rely on what they say, we can rely on what they do—which version of shrimp coconut jambalaya they polished off.

But on one dark Thursday night in the first week of February 2004, something a little more mischievous was planned for diners who braved the snow to keep their reservations. They were getting a full glass of Cabernet Sauvignon before their meal. Totally free. Compliments of the house.

This cabernet was not a fine vintage. In fact, it was a $2 bottle sold under the brand name Charles Shaw—popularly known as Two Buck Chuck. But our diners didn't know this. In fact, all the Charles Shaw labels had been soaked off the bottles and replaced with professionally designed labels that were 100 percent fake.

Those on the left side of the room were being offered wine from the fictional Noah's Winery, a new California label. The winery's classic, italicized logo was enveloped by a simple graphic of grapes and vines. Below this, the wine proudly announced that it was "NEW from California." After the diners arrived and were seated, the waiter or waitress said, "Good evening and welcome to the Spice Box. As you're deciding what you want to eat this evening, we're offering you a complimentary glass of Cabernet Sauvignon. It's from a new California winery called Noah's Winery." Each person was then poured a standard 3.8-ounce glass of wine.[4]

About an hour later, after they had finished their meal and were paying for it, we weighed the amount of wine left in each glass and the amount of the entrée left on each plate. We also had a record of when each diner had started eating and when they paid their bill and left.

Diners on the right side of the room had exactly the same dining experience—with one exception. The waiter or waitress's carefully scripted welcome introduced a cabernet "from a new *North Dakota* winery called Noah's Winery." The label was identical to that on the first bottle, except for the words "NEW from North Dakota."

There is no Bordeaux region in North Dakota, nor is there a Burgundy region, nor a Champagne region. There is, however, a Fargo region, a Bismarck region, and a Minot region. It's just that there are no wine grapes grown in any of them. California equals wine. North Dakota equals snow or buffalo.

People who were given "North Dakota wine" believed it *was* North Dakota wine. But since it was the same wine we poured for those who thought they were getting California wine, that shouldn't influence their taste. Should it?

It did. We knew from an earlier lab study that people

who thought they were drinking North Dakota wine had such low expectations, they rated the wine as tasting bad *and* their food as less tasty. If a California wine label can give a glowing halo to an entire meal, a North Dakota wine label casts a shadow onto everything it touches.

But our focus that particular night was whether these labels would influence *how much* our diners ate.

After the meals were over, the first thing we discovered was that both groups of people drank about the same amount of wine—all of it. This was not so surprising. It was only one glass of wine and it was a cold night. Where they differed was in how much food they ate and how long they lingered at their table.

Compared to those unlucky diners given wine with North Dakota labels, people who thought they had been given a free glass of California wine ate 11 percent more of their food—19 of the 24 even cleaned their plates. They also lingered an average of 10 minutes longer at their table (64 minutes). They stayed pretty much until the waitstaff starting dropping hints that the next seating would be starting soon.

The night was not quite as magical for those given wine with the North Dakota label. Not only did they leave more food on their plates, this probably wasn't much of a meal to remember, because it went by so fast. North Dakota wine drinkers sat down, drank, ate, paid, and were out in 55 minutes—less than an hour. For them, this was clearly not a special meal, it was just food.

Exact same meals, exact same wine. Different labels, different reactions.

Now, to a cold-eyed skeptic, there should have been no difference between the two groups. They should have eaten the same amount and enjoyed it the same.

They didn't. *They mindlessly ate.* That is, once they were given a free glass of "California" wine, they said to themselves: "This is going to be good." Once they concluded it was going to be good, their experience lined up to confirm their expectations. They no longer had to stop and think about whether the food and wine were really as good as they thought. They had already decided.

Of course, the same thing happened to the diners who were given the "North Dakota" wine. Once they saw the label, they set themselves up for disappointment. There was no halo; there was a shadow. And not only was the wine bad, the entire meal fell short.

After our studies are over, we "debrief" people—often by e-mail—and tell them what the study was about and what results we expect. For instance, with our different wine studies, we might say, "We think the average person drinking what they believe is North Dakota wine will like their meal less than those given the 'California' wine." We then ask the kicker: "Do you think you were influenced by the state's name you saw on the label?" Almost all will give the exact same answer: "No, I wasn't."

In the thousands of debriefings we've done for hundreds of studies, nearly every person who was "tricked" by the words on a label, the size of a package, the lighting in a room, or the size of a plate said, "I wasn't influenced by that."

They might acknowledge that others could be "fooled," but they don't think *they* were. That is what gives mindless eating so much power over us—we're not aware it's happening.

Even when we *do* pay close attention we are suggestible—and even when it comes to cold, hard numbers. Take the concept of anchoring. If you ask people if there are more or less than 50 calories in an apple, most will say more. When you ask them how many, the average person will say, "66." If you had instead asked if there were more or less than 150 calories in an apple, most would say less. When you ask them how many, the average person would say, "114." People unknowingly anchor or focus on the number they first hear and let that bias them.

A while back, I teamed up with two professor friends of mine—Steve Hoch and Bob Kent—to see if anchoring influences how much food we buy in grocery stores. We believed that grocery shoppers who saw numerical signs such as "Limit 12 Per Person" would buy much more than those who saw signs such as "No Limit Per Person." To nail down the psychology behind this, we repeated this study in different forms, using different numbers, different promotions (like "2 for $2" versus "1 for $1"), and in different supermarkets and convenience stores. By the time we finished, we knew that almost *any* sign with a number promotion leads us to buy 30 to 100 percent more than we normally would.[5]

After the research was completed and published in the *Journal of Marketing Research*, another friend and I were in the checkout line at a grocery store, where I saw a sign advertising gum, "10 packs for $2." I was eagerly counting out 10 packs onto the conveyer belt, when my friend commented, "Didn't you just publish a big research paper on that?"

We're *all* tricked by our environment. Even if we "know it" in our head, most of the time we have way too much on our mind to remember it and act on it. That's why it's easier to change our environment than our mind.

The Dieter's Dilemma

We've all heard of somebody's cousin's sister who went on a huge diet before her high school reunion, lost tons of weight, kept it off, won the lottery, and lived happily ever after. Yet we also know about 95 times as many people who started a diet and gave up in discouragement, or who started a diet, lost weight, gained more weight, and *then* gave up in discouragement.[6] After that, they started a different diet and repeated the same depriving, discouraging, demoralizing process. Indeed, it's estimated that over 95 percent of all people who lose weight on a diet gain it back.[7]

Most diets are deprivation diets. We deprive ourselves or deny ourselves of something—carbohydrates, fat, red meat, snacks, pizza, breakfast, chocolate, and so forth. Unfortunately, deprivation diets don't work for three reasons: 1) Our body fights against them; 2) our brain fights against them; and 3) our day-to-day environment fights against them.

Millions of years of evolution have made our body too smart to fall for our little "I'm only eating salad" trick. Our body's metabolism is efficient. When it has plenty of food to burn, it turns up the furnace and burns our fat reserves faster. When it has less food to burn, it turns down the furnace and burns it more slowly and efficiently. This efficiency helped our ancestors survive famines and barren winters.

Deprivation Diets and the Academy Awards:
Pounds That Are Here, Gone, and Back Again Next Week

You know how it is. One day you're mindlessly eating ice cream in front of an open freezer door and—*bam*—all of a sudden you remember you have to be at the Academy Awards ceremony in three days.

How do the movie stars lose those last-minute pounds before walking the runway at the Oscars? An article in *People* showed that what they usually do is drastic, painful—and temporary.[8]

- EMMA THOMPSON: I try not to eat sugar, and I don't eat bread and biscuits. Actually, to be frank, I really don't eat any of the things I love, which is unfortunate. But I will get back to ice cream soon, which is my favorite food.
- TARA REID: I won't eat that morning and that week I will only eat protein—egg whites and chicken. It makes a big difference. You look hot for a week, but you gain it all back the next. I also drink way more water.
- VIVICA A. FOX: I pop herbal laxatives and drink as much coffee as I can to flush everything out.
- MELISSA RIVERS: I limit my calorie intake and work out like crazy. I try to eat really clean the week prior. I always substitute one meal for just a salad with dressing on the side, and I dip my fork in the dressing.
- BILL MURRAY: I did 200,000 crunches.

Drastic? Yes. Successful? As you can see from their answers, these deprivation diets worked only as long as was absolutely necessary. Five minutes after the Academy Awards ceremony is over, it's back to the normal routine, and the 10 pounds that were lost begin to find their way home again. Unless you're not yet finished with your 200,000 crunches.

But it doesn't help today's deprived dieter. If you eat too little, the body goes into conservation mode and makes it even tougher to burn off the pounds.

This type of weight loss is not mindless. It's like pushing a boulder uphill every second of every day.

How much weight loss triggers the conservation switch? It seems that we can lose half a pound a week without triggering a metabolism slowdown.[9] Some people may be able to lose more, but everyone can lose at least half a pound a week and still be in full-burn mode. The only problem is that this is too slow for many of us. We think weight loss has to be all or nothing. This is why so many impatient people try to lose it all and end up losing nothing.

Now for our brains. If we consciously deny ourselves something again and again, we're likely to end up craving it more and more.[10]

It doesn't matter whether you're deprived of affection, vacation, television, or your favorite foods. Being deprived is not a great way to enjoy life. Nevertheless, the first thing many dieters do is cut out their comfort foods. This becomes a recipe for dieting disaster, because any diet that is based on denying yourself the foods you really like is going to be really temporary. The foods we don't bite can come back to bite us. When the diet ends—either because of frustration or because of temporary success—you're back wolfing down your comfort foods with a hungry vengeance. With all that sacrificing you've been doing, there's a lot of catching up to do.

When it comes to losing weight, we can't rely only on our brain, or our "cognitive control," a.k.a. willpower. If we're making more than 200 food-related decisions each day,

The Bigger the Deprivation,
the Bigger the Fall

". . . a nationally known psychologist and expert on eating disorders was arrested in a West Hartford, Conn., convenience store after, according to police, passing out from inhaling the aerosol from three cans of whipped cream."

—"News of the Weird," October 2005[11]

as our research has shown, it's almost impossible to have them all be diet-book perfect. We have millions of years of evolution and instinct telling us to eat as often as we can and to eat as much as we can. Most of us simply do not have the mental fortitude to stare at a plate of warm cookies on the table and say, "I'm not going to eat a cookie, I'm not going to eat a cookie," and then not eat the cookie. It's only so long before our "No, no, maybe, maybe" turns into a "Yes."

Our bodies fight against deprivation, and our brains fight against deprivation.[12] And to make matters worse, our day-to-day environment is set up to booby-trap any half-hearted effort we can muster. There are great smells on every fast-food corner. There are warm, comfort-food feelings we get from television commercials. There are better-than-homemade-tasting 85¢ snacks in every vending machine and gas station. We have billions of dollars' worth of marketing giving us the perfect foods that our big hearts and big tummies desire.

Yet before we blame those evil marketers, let's look at the traps we set for ourselves. We make an extra "family-size" portion of pasta so no one goes hungry at dinner. We lovingly leave latchkey snacks on the table for our children (and ourselves). We use the nice, platter-size dinner plates that we can pile with food. We heat up a piece of apple pie in the microwave while the lonely apple shivers in the crisper. Best intentions aside, we're Public Enemy #1 when it comes to booby-trapping the diets and willpower of both ourselves and our family.

The good news is that the same levers that almost invisibly lead you to slowly gain weight can also be pushed in the other direction to just as invisibly lead you to slowly lose weight—*unknowingly.* If we don't realize we're eating a little less than we need, we don't feel deprived. If we don't feel deprived, we're less likely to backslide and find ourselves overeating to compensate for everything we've forgone. The key lies in the *mindless margin*.

The Mindless Margin

No one goes to bed skinny and wakes up fat. Most people gain (or lose) weight so gradually they can't really figure out how it happened. They don't remember changing their eating or exercise patterns.[13] All they remember is once being able to fit into their favorite pants without having to hold their breath and hope they can get the zipper to budge.

Sure, there are exceptions. If we gorge ourselves at the all-you-can-eat pizza buffet, then clean out the chip bowl at the Super Bowl party, then stop by the Baskin-Robbins drive-through for a belly-buster sundae on the way home, we realize we've gone too far over the top. But on most days we have very little idea whether we've eaten 50 calories too much or 50 calories too little. In fact, most of us wouldn't know if we ate 200 or 300 calories more or less than the day before.

This is the mindless margin. It's the margin or zone in which we can either slightly overeat or slightly undereat without being aware of it. Suppose you can eat 2,000 calories a day without either gaining or losing weight.[14] If one day, however, you only ate 1,000 calories, you would know it. You'd feel weak, light-headed, cranky, and you'd snap at the dog. On the other hand, you'd also know it if you ate 3,000 calories. You'd feel a little heavier, slower, and more like flopping on the couch and petting the cat.

If we eat way too little, we know it. If we eat way too much, we know it. But there is a calorie range—*a mindless margin*—where we feel fine and are unaware of small differences. That is, the difference between 1,900 calories and 2,000 calories is one we cannot detect, nor can we detect the difference between 2,000 and 2,100 calories. But over the course of a year, this mindless margin would either cause us to lose ten pounds or to gain ten pounds. It takes 3,500 extra calories to equal one pound. It doesn't matter if we eat these extra 3,500 calories in one week or gradually over the entire year. They'll add up to one pound.

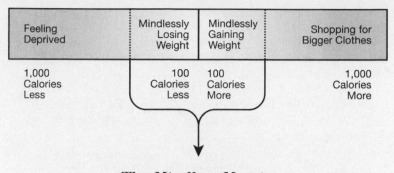

Feeling Deprived	Mindlessly Losing Weight	Mindlessly Gaining Weight	Shopping for Bigger Clothes
1,000 Calories Less	100 Calories Less	100 Calories More	1,000 Calories More

The Mindless Margin

This is the danger of creeping calories. Just 10 extra calories a day—one stick of Doublemint gum or three small Jelly Belly jelly beans—will make you a pound more portly one year from today.[15] Only three Jelly Bellys a day.

Fortunately, the same thing happens in the opposite direction.

One colleague of mine, Cindy, had lost around 20 pounds during her first two years at a new job. When I asked how she lost the weight, she couldn't really answer. After some persistent questioning, it seemed that the only deliberate change she'd made two years earlier was to give up caffeine. She switched from coffee to herbal tea. That didn't seem to explain anything.

"Oh yeah," she said, "and because I gave up caffeine, I also stopped drinking Coke." She had been drinking about six cans a week—far from a serious habit—but the 139 calories in each Coke translated into 12 pounds a year. She wasn't even aware of why she'd lost weight. In her mind all she'd done was cut out caffeine.

In a classic article in *Science,* Drs. James O. Hill and John C. Peters suggested that cutting only 100 calories a

How Much Will I Lose in a Year?

If you make a change, there's an easy way to estimate how much weight you'll lose in a year. You simply divide the calories by 10. That's roughly the number of pounds you'll lose if you're otherwise in energy balance.

One less 270 calorie candy bar each day = 27 fewer pounds a year
One less 140 calorie soft drink each day = 14 fewer pounds a year
One less 420 calorie bagel or donut each day = 42 fewer pounds a year

The same thing works with burning calories: walking one extra mile a day is 100 calories and 10 pounds a year. Exercise is good, but for most people it's a lot easier to give up a candy bar than to walk 2.7 miles to a vending machine.

day from our diets would prevent weight gain in most of the U.S. population.[16] If the majority of people gain only a pound or two each year, anything a person does to make this 100-calorie difference will lead most of us to *lose* weight. We can do it by walking an extra 2,000 steps each day (about one mile), or we can do it by eating 100 calories less than we otherwise would.

The best way to trim 100 or 200 calories a day is to do it in a way that doesn't make you feel deprived. It's easy to re-arrange your kitchen and change a few eating habits so you don't have to think about eating less or differently. And the silver lining is that the same things that lead us to mind-lessly gain weight can also help us mindlessly lose weight.

How much weight? Unlike what you hear in 3:00 A.M. infomercials, it would not be 10 pounds in 10 hours, or 10 pounds in 10 days. It's not even going to be 10 pounds in 10 weeks. You would notice that, and you would feel deprived. Instead, suppose you stay within the mindless margin for losing weight and trim 100–200 calories a day. You probably won't feel deprived, and in 10 months you'll be in the neighborhood of 10 pounds lighter. It won't put you in this year's *Sports Illustrated* swimsuit issue, but it might put you back in some of your "signal" clothes, and it'll make you feel better without costing you bread, pasta, and your comfort foods.

Cutting out our favorite foods is a bad idea. Cutting down on *how much* of them we eat is mindlessly do-able. Many fad diets focus more on the *types* of foods we can eat rather than *how much* we should eat. But the problem isn't that we order beef instead of a low-fat chicken breast. The problem is that the beef is often twice the size. A low-fat chicken breast that we resent having to eat may be no better for our long-term diet than a tastier but slightly smaller piece of beef.

If we're looking at only a 100- or 200-calorie difference a day, these are not calories we'll miss. We can trim them out of our day relatively easily—and unknowingly. Herein lies the secret of the mindless margin.

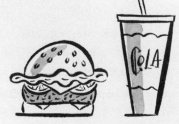

"I'm Not Hungry but I'm Going to Eat This Anyway."

Over coffee, a new friend commented that he'd lost 30 pounds within the past year. When I asked him how, he explained he didn't stop eating potato chips, pizza, or ice cream. He ate anything he wanted, but if he had a craving when he wasn't hungry he'd say— out loud—"I'm not hungry but I'm going to eat this anyway."

Having to make that declaration—out loud—would often be enough to prevent him from mindlessly indulging. Other times, he would take a nibble but be much more mindful of what he was doing.

Reengineering Strategy #1:
Think 20 Percent–More or Less

While most Americans stop eating when they're full, those in leaner cultures stop eating when they're no longer hungry. There's a significant calorie gap between the point where an Okinawan says, "I'm no longer hungry," and where an American says, "I'm full." The Okinawans even have an expression for when to stop eating. They call the concept *hara hachi bu*—eating until you're just 80 percent full.[17]

- **Think 20 percent less.** Dish out 20 percent less than you think you might want before you start to eat. You probably won't miss it. In most of our studies, people can eat 20 percent less without noticing it. If they eat 30 percent less they realize it, but 20 percent is still under the radar screen.

• **For fruits and vegetables, think 20 percent more.** If you cut down how much pasta you dish out by 20 percent, increase the veggies by 20 percent.

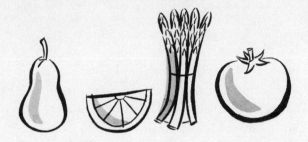

2

The Forgotten Food

YOUR STOMACH CAN'T COUNT.
It can't count the number of spoonfuls of Golden Grahams you had for breakfast. It can't count the number of ounces in the overpriced Frappuccino you drank on the way to work. It can't count the number of French fries you inhaled in the first 90 seconds of your lunch. It can't count the number of calories in the aptly named Chubby Hubby ice cream you ate standing in front of the refrigerator when you got home.

Our stomachs are bad at math, and what's more, we get no help from our attention or our memory. We don't register how many pieces of candy we had from the communal candy dish at work, and whether we ate 20 French fries or 30. It gets even worse when we're out dining with our friends and family. Five minutes after dinner, 31 percent of the people leaving an Italian restaurant couldn't even remember how much bread they ate, and 12 percent of the bread eaters denied having eaten any bread at all.[1]

Considering our imperfect food memory, it seems that the last person we should rely on to stop eating is ourselves. It's not necessarily that we're trying to fool ourselves, or that we're living in blissful, snug-clothing denial. We're just not designed to accurately keep track of how much we've consumed.[2]

If we could see what we've eaten, we would probably eat less. For instance, if we could see *all* of the Chinese food we shoveled onto our buffet plates, or if we could see *all* of the handfuls of potato chips we've already inhaled before reaching for another, we would probably stop eating before the point where our stomach hurts.

Unfortunately, most foods don't leave a table trace. That is, after we eat them, all evidence is gone; all that remains is an empty plate. Chicken wings—now known by sports-bar sophisticates as "Buffalo wings"—are different. After we finish a chicken wing, the bony evidence remains. If we eat three chicken wings, we see three bones. If we eat eight chicken wings, we see eight bones.

This gave my graduate students and me an idea. Usually when people are given all of the chicken wings they can eat—such as at a party or at a sports bar—the bones are continuously bussed from the table and we lose track of how many we've eaten. What would happen if the bones stayed right there? Every time the partygoers looked down, there would be a stark reminder—a running, boney count. Would this lead them to eat less?

On one Super Bowl Sunday, we invited 53 MBA students to a party at a local sports bar to test our idea. We promised them free chicken wings, a big screen, and a great excuse to avoid studying.

Super Bowls and Super Food

The Super Bowl means big calorie business. Here's the tally, as reported by *USA Today:*[3]

1st—Where the Super Bowl ranks in terms of home parties. It even beats New Year's Eve.
2nd—Where the Super Bowl ranks in food consumption.
17—The average number of partiers at each Super Bowl party.
68—The percentage of partiers who prefer pizza as their game-day meal.
4,000—The tons of popcorn people will eat.
14,000—The tons of chips they will eat.
3,200,000—The number of pizzas Pizza Hut and Domino's expected to sell during the 2005 Super Bowl.

When the hungry MBA students arrived, they were led into a private party area and seated on bar stools at the high, four-person tables. In the center of the room was the "Buffalo Buffet"—loaded with heaping steam trays of wings and a number of sauces that looked like scalding Cheez Whiz or scorched low-price BBQ sauce. After ordering what they wanted to drink (soft drinks were free), the students circled the buffet and pounced. They took all the wings they wanted and returned to their tables. When they finished their chicken wings, they could pile up the bones in the empty bowls that were conveniently provided on each table.

Throughout the evening, whenever they wanted more

wings, all they had to do was roll off their bar stool and amble over to the Buffalo Buffet. Every time the Super Bowl commercials came on, they could disrespectfully ignore millions of dollars' worth of advertising genius and go refill their plates.

The waitresses were working with us, and they were instructed to bus the leftover chicken bones from only half of the tables. They bussed these tables three or four times through the night, each time leaving a clean, empty bowl for future bones. While the waitresses were out front, we were in the kitchen. When they brought the bones back to the kitchen, they told us which table each bowl came from. We then counted (and weighed) the number of leftover bones to determine how much the people at that table had eaten.

But that's only half the story. The waitresses had also been instructed to ignore the growing piles of bones on the other tables. They could stop by and take drink orders, but the bones just kept piling up where they lay. After the game was over and the happy MBA students had left the building, we went over to these tables, counted the bones, weighed them, and rolled the garbage cans over.

Sometimes it even surprises us how predictable people are. If our guests had their tables continually bussed, they continually ate. Clean plate, clean table, get more, eat more. Their stomachs could not count, so the clear-table group kept eating until they thought they were full. They ate an average of seven chicken wings apiece.

The people at the bone-pile tables were less of a threat to the chicken population. After the Super Bowl was over, they had eaten an average of two fewer chicken wings per person—28 percent less than those whose tables had been bussed.[4]

Our stomach can't count and we don't remember. Unless we can actually see what we're eating, we can very easily overeat. Unless a person consistently weighs him- or herself, most people start realizing they've overeaten (and have gained weight) only when their clothing gets uncomfortably tight.

Some people have to go to jail to learn this lesson.

The Prison Pounds Mystery

The food served in county jails is not typically awarded any Michelin stars. In fact, complaining about the food is one of the great inmate pastimes. This is why a sheriff at one Midwestern jail was puzzled when he noticed an odd trend: The inmates, with an average sentence of six months, were mysteriously gaining 20–25 "prison pounds" during the course of their "visit." It wasn't because the food was great. Nor did it seem to be because they hadn't exercised or because they were lonely or bored. They generally had access to exercise facilities and to daily visitors.

In fact, upon release, no inmate blamed the food, the exercise machines, or the visitation hours for their weight gain. They blamed their jailhouse fat on the baggy orange jumpsuits they had to wear for six months. Because these orange coveralls were so loose-fitting, most of them didn't realize they had progressively gained weight—about a pound a week—until they were released and had to try and squeeze back into their own clothes.[5]

Most of us don't wake up after six months and discover

"Does This Orange Jumpsuit Make Me Look Fat?"

No one will say, "Yes, it makes you look like a large, orange highway cone that can be seen from the planet Pluto." The answer you'll get, of course, is, "Oh, no, you look just fine." Instead of asking someone else's opinion, here are two rough rules of thumb you can use to figure out whether your weight is on track. These are not exact, but they'll give you a good idea of where you stand.

- **The BMI Rule of Thumb:** BMI stands for Body Mass Index, and it's what scientists and doctors use to determine if someone is overweight. Since it's based on the metric system, we need to use an extra step if using pounds and feet. First, you take your weight in pounds and divide it by the square of your height in inches. Then multiply this number by 703.

  What's a good BMI? Normal is 18.5–24.9; 25–29.9 is overweight; 30+ is obese.[6]

  So, if a person is 5'8" and 180 pounds, their BMI would be 27.4 [(180 pounds / 68x68) x 703 = 27.4]. That would classify this person as overweight.

- **The Body Frame Rule of Thumb:** This is for ladies only. Some modeling and acting coaches use this rule of thumb to help women picture their ideal runway weight. Allow 100 pounds for the first five feet of your height and five pounds for each additional inch. Then, if you have a small frame, subtract 10 pounds. If you have a medium frame, add zero; if you have a big frame, add 10.[7]

  For a big-boned woman who is 5'3", this works out to 125 pounds [100 + (3x5) + 10 = 125]. A medium-framed woman who is 5'6" should be about 130 pounds [100 + (6x5) + 0 = 130].

that we're 25 pounds heavier. Why? Partly because we don't wear highway-cone orange jumpsuits day in and day out. If we gain 10 pounds, that really nice pair of dress slacks only zips up halfway. If we gain 20 pounds, our belt runs out of notches and we have to use rope. Just as we can't tell how much we've eaten simply by relying on internal cues, we can't really tell how much we've gained or lost without some external benchmark.

A surprising number of people don't use a scale to monitor their weight, but they do use other sorts of signals. My Lab asked 322 dieters how they would know they had lost the right amount of weight if they didn't have a scale. Many pointed toward external cues. Some said that regardless of what their scale said, they would know they had lost enough weight when they got compliments from friends or "second looks" from strangers. Others said they would know it when they could "see it"—"it" being things like cheekbones, ribs, their feet, and so forth.

Most of these dieters—over half—pointed at their clothes. They knew they would be at the weight they wanted when they got down to a certain belt notch, or when they didn't have to inhale to button their pants, or when they could comfortably sit down in their old jeans without losing blood circulation in their legs.

Our clothes don't lie. They fit, or they don't fit. For some people, losing 20 pounds is an abstract concept. But being able to fit into their favorite jeans is not at all abstract. To dieters, such clothes are called "signal clothes." When they fit, they signal that it's fine to stop eating rice cakes at every meal.

The Top 8 Signals People Use
to Know They've Lost Weight

Other than staring at the bathroom scale, what are the most common signals people use to know they're at the right weight? Here's what 322 people told us in a recent survey:

- "When my jeans feel comfortable again."
- "When I have to start wearing a belt."
- "When I suck in my stomach, and I can see some definition, like a four-pack."
- "When my belt notch moves back to where it used to be."
- "When I don't get tired walking up two flights of stairs to my office."
- "When I can see my cheekbones."
- "When I don't have to inhale to button my pants."
- "When friends or colleagues ask me if I've lost weight."

We Believe Our Eyes, Not Our Stomach

Over time, our clothes may tell us that we've overeaten, but how do we know if we're having too much when we're smack in the middle of dinner? Short of eating until it hurts, most of us seem to rely on the size—the volume—of the food to tell us when we're full. We usually try to eat the same visible amount of food we're used to eating. That is, we want to eat the same size lunch that we did yesterday, the same size dinner, the same size of popcorn, and so on. This ends up actually being an advantage, because it holds a key to painlessly eating less.

One of the most honest and helpful diet books of the last decade was *The Volumetrics Eating Plan*,[8] by Dr. Barbara Rolls of the Center for Behavioral Nutrition at Penn State. It's based on thousands of hours of meticulous lab studies that show—like our Food and Brand Lab studies—that we're pretty much clueless about when we've had enough to eat. While it's hard to calculate calories, it's easy to eyeball a portion size. We know that we'll be full if we eat a full plate of food, and we'll be half-full if we eat only a half plate of food. We know that if we eat a hamburger that takes two hands to hold, we should be full. But if we eat one that we can easily hold with a thumb and two fingers, we'll be looking around for more.

So if somebody typically eats a huge half-pound ham-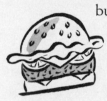burger, and you give them a quarter-pound hamburger, they'll eat it and still feel hungry. Rolls found, however, that if you make the quarter-pound hamburger *look* the same size as the half-pound hamburger, by adding lettuce, tomato, onion, and not squishing it down before serving it, the same hungry person will eat it and say he's full. Even though it has many fewer calories than the half-pound burger, people will still rate themselves as equally full after lunch is over. Although this was puzzling news to scientists dealing with physiology and metabolism, it was great news to dieters. It meant they could cut the size of their meat and cheese in half, and as long as they added enough garden greens to make the hamburger look just as big, they'd feel as full as if they'd eaten the real deal.[9]

In one demonstration, Rolls' team made a small amount

of food look big simply by adding air to it. They took the exact same strawberry smoothie ingredients and put them in the blender for different amounts of time. The longer in the blender, the more air got whipped into the smoothie, and the bigger it looked. They could start with a smoothie that filled only half a glass, and if they blended it long enough, it would fill up the entire glass.

They then gave these half-glass and full-glass smoothies to some male college students 30 minutes before lunch. Both smoothies had exactly the same number of calories. All that differed was their size. Those students who were given the full glasses ended up eating 12 percent less lunch. They also claimed to feel more full.

Scores of studies have shown that we typically eat about the same amount or volume of food each day, and even at each meal. Rolls' work emphasizes that if a person *thinks* he ate less than that typical volume, he'll think he's hungry. If he thinks he ate more, he'll think he's full.

In other words, volume trumps calories. We eat the *volume* we want, not the calories we want. If you were to make a given amount of food twice as caloric, people wouldn't complain that they couldn't eat all of it. If you made the same amount half as caloric, people wouldn't complain they were still hungry. In both cases, they would say they were full. People don't eat calories, they eat volume.[10]

There's a saying in the food industry that the two cheapest ingredients you can add to food are water and air. Not a bad idea to remember.

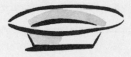

Eye It, Dish It, Eat It

We stop eating when our stomach is full, right?

Oddly enough, this is wrong. We don't stop eating because our stomach is full except in very extreme cases, such as Thanksgiving dinner. In reality, scientists don't know exactly what makes us feel full. It seems to be a combination, among other things, of how much we chew, how much we taste, how much we swallow, how much we think about the food, and how long we have been eating.

What does seem to be the case is that the faster we wolf down our food, the more we eat, because this combination of cues doesn't get the chance to tell us we're no longer hungry. Many research studies show that it takes up to 20 minutes for our body and brain to signal satiation, so that we realize we are full. Twenty minutes is enough time to inhale two or three more pieces of pizza and chug a large refill of Pepsi.

Here's the problem. We Americans start, finish, and clear the table for many of our meals in *less* than 20 minutes. Our meals are remarkably short. Take lunch, for example. Drs. Rick Bell and Patti Pliner found that if we're eating lunch alone, we spend only 11 minutes eating if we're at a fast-food restaurant, 13 minutes at a workplace cafeteria, and 28 minutes at a moderately priced restaurant. If we're eating with three other people, we tend to eat about twice as long, but that's still a speedy lunch.[11]

Most of us actually decide how much to eat *before* we put any food into our mouths. We eyeball how much we think we want, dish it out, and then eat until it's gone. That is, after we say, "I want two scoops of ice cream" or "half a bowl of soup," we rely on that visual cue—the empty ice cream bowl or the half-empty soup bowl—to tell us we're through.

Think of a jogger. If she decides to jog on a treadmill until she's tired, she constantly has to ask herself, "Am I tired yet, am I tired yet, am I tired yet?" But if she says, "I'm going to jog down to the school and back," she doesn't have to constantly monitor how tired she is. She sets the target, and jogs until she's done.

This is one reason why the "clean your plate" notion is so powerful. The clean plate gives us a set target to aim for so we don't have to constantly ask ourselves, "Am I full yet, am I full yet, am I full yet?" We can dish it out, space out, and eat until it's gone.

The Bottomless Soup Bowl

We showed a number of American college students an 18-ounce bowl of tomato soup and asked them, "If you were going to have this soup for lunch, when would you decide to stop eating?" Eighty-one percent gave a visual reference point, such as "I'd stop when the bowl was empty" or "I'd eat half of it." Only 19 percent said they would decide to stop eating when they were full or no longer hungry. In this case, it seems like most of these people eyeballed how much they thought they would eat and then, like the jogger running to the school and back, they pretty much planned to keep eating until they had a visual cue that it was time to stop. But what happens if the plate is never clean, or the bowl never empties?

Your Stomach's Three Settings

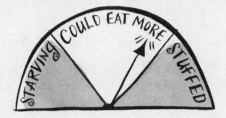

In the hundreds of studies we've done on food, it became increasingly clear that the stomach only has three main settings:

1) Starving
2) I'm Full but I Can Eat More
3) I'm Stuffed

There's a bottom level, or floor, where you feel equally hungry whether you haven't eaten for 8 hours or for 18 hours. There's a top level, or ceiling, beyond which you can't continue to eat. In between is the gray zone where you can always eat more—even when you're close to the ceiling. Remember how many Thanksgiving dinners you felt almost sickeningly full? Remember that when the dessert was served, more room in your stomach magically appeared? This is why we need to focus on the setting "I'm Full but I Can Eat More." This is the level where we can cut our mindless margin and still be satisfied.

Jim Painter, Jill North, and I devised a *Candid Camera*–like experiment to find out.

Although you would never find the construction plans for bottomless soup bowls in the back of *Popular Mechanics,*

here's how they're made. You take a sturdy, four-person restaurant table, check that the restaurant owner isn't around,
and drill a big one-inch hole right through the table where
a waiter would ordinarily set a soup bowl. (A better option
is to buy the table and *then* drill the hole.)

Then you drill another hole in the bottom of a soup
bowl so that you can attach food-grade rubber tubing to it.
You poke the other end of the tubing through the hole in
the table, duct-tape it to the underside, and run it over to a
six-quart pot of hot soup. If you place the pot of soup at the
right height, a person can eat out of that soup bowl all day
and it will automatically keep refilling itself. It won't refill
itself back to the top of the bowl, so people will believe
they're making progress even though the bowl never com-
pletely empties. It's all physics: atmospheric pressure keeps
the liquid in the 18-ounce bowl at the same height as it
keeps the liquid in the 6-quart soup vat. The fill level in both
drops at the same rate.

Our table seated four people. Two had their refillable
bowls rigged up to separate six-quart soup vats, and the
other two had normal bowls that looked identical. This might
sound straightforward, but the practice trials were disasters.
There were four kinks that needed to be ironed out:

1. **The Tube.** When a tube pokes up into their soup bowl,
   lunchgoers tend to get suspicious. With the help of a me-
   chanical engineering student, a brass "bayonet mount"
   was fitted to the bottom of the bowl, so the refilling tube
   couldn't be detected by running your spoon over it.
2. **The Bowl.** What if someone tried to move their bowl?
   Since our participants were good Midwesterners, this

problem was solved simply by asking them to not touch their bowls so we could "keep everything organized and consistent." Whatever that meant, it worked.

3. **The Story.** People kept trying to guess why they were getting a free lunch. They were always wrong, but we were afraid that their guessing game would keep them from eating normally. So we told them that in exchange for lunch we would ask them a few questions about their impression of the college cafeteria and the quality of food it offered. We also moved the study to the Spice Box, where they knew recipes were often tested.

4. **The Soup.** Our bottomless bowls failed to function during the first practice trial. The chicken noodle soup we were using either clogged the tubes or caused the soup to gurgle strangely. We bought 360 quarts of Campbell's tomato soup, and started over.

Once we ironed out the kinks, we recruited more than 60 people for a soup lunch. Each day four were seated together at a table—two had 18-ounce refillable soup bowls and the other two had normal 18-ounce soup bowls that were filled all the way to the top.

You might think that if you were asked to join three semi-strangers at a table for lunch, there might be some uncomfortable moments. Not so with college students. All we had to do was ask them what their plans were for the summer, and the conversation flowed as fast as the soup.

After 20 minutes, we stopped the study and asked our lunchgoers to estimate how many calories they had eaten, how many ounces of soup they had eaten, and how full they were on a 9-point scale. The soup was then drained from the bowls, tubes, and pots, and it was weighed to figure out exactly how much each one had slurped.

Of the 62 people who showed up for lunch, only two discovered what was occurring. One bent down to retrieve a dropped napkin, and quickly pointed out the Borg-like tubing under the table to the rest of his lunch companions. The second person had a much more dramatic experience. Forgetting for a moment that he was not at a medieval banquet, this man picked up his bowl to drink out of it as if he were channeling one of his Viking ancestors. It made a loud gurgle and the tomato soup–filled tube slithered up through the table like a coral snake. This made the woman next to him shriek, and the man across from him tipped over his chair in his haste to escape. These two people and their companions were dropped from the study. None of the other 54 suspected a thing.

People eating out of the normal soup bowls ate about 9

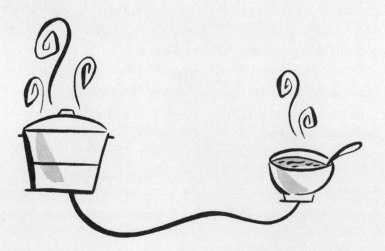

ounces of soup. This is just a little less than the size of a nondiluted Campbell's soup can (10.5 ounces). They thought they had eaten about 123 calories' worth of soup, but, in fact, they had eaten 155. People eating out of the bottomless soup bowls ate and ate and ate. Most were still eating when we stopped them, 20 minutes after they began. The typical person ate around 15 ounces, but others ate more than a quart—*more than a quart.* When one of these people was asked to comment on the soup, his reply was, "It's pretty good, and it's pretty filling." Sure it is. He had eaten almost three times as much as the guy sitting next to him.[12]

Surely diners realized that they ate more from the refillable bowl? Absolutely not. With a couple of exceptions, such as Mr. Quart Man, people didn't comment about feeling full. Even though they ate 73 percent more, they rated themselves the same as the others—after all, they only had about half a bowl of soup. Or so they thought. When asked how many calories of soup they ate, the 127 calories they estimated was nearly the same as that estimated by those people eating from the normal bowls. In reality, they had eaten an average of 268 calories. This was 113 calories more than their tablemates with the normal bowls.

Not knowing when to stop turns Thanksgiving dinners, buffets, and dim sum restaurants into diet dangers. And what if we earnestly try to guesstimate how many calories we're eating? Sorry, it still won't help much.

Why French Women Don't Get Fat

Why don't French women get fat—even though they consume cheese, baguettes, wine, pastries, and pâté? As Mireille Guiliano proposed in her bestselling book, it is because they know when to stop eating. Our own research suggests that they pay more attention to internal clues, such as whether they feel full, and less attention to the external clues (like the level of soup in a bowl) that can lead us to overeat.

To see if this was true, we had 282 Parisians and Chicagoans fill out questionnaires asking them how they decided it was time to stop eating a meal. Parisians reported that they usually stopped eating when they no longer felt hungry. Not our Chicagoans. They stopped when they ran out of a beverage, or when their plate was empty, or when the television show they were watching was over. Yet the heavier a person was—American or French—the more they relied on external cues to tell them when to stop eating and the less they relied on whether they felt full.[13]

People-Size or Meal-Size?

Our experience with thousands of people suggests that most of us are terrible at estimating how many calories we have eaten so far today, or yesterday, or last week. On average, normal weight people think they've eaten 20 percent less than they actually did. Those three pieces of pizza you thought were 1,000 calories were actually 1,250, and that 200-calorie donut was actually 250. But the real concern is with obese people. They typically underestimate how much they eat by 30 to 40 percent. Some think they eat *half* as much as they actually do.[14]

This has been a mystery. Scientists, physicians, and counselors have often blamed overweight people for trying to fool others (or themselves) about how much they're eating. Some dieticians, physicians, and family members tell them flat out that they're "lying" or "in denial." Hurtful accusations like these only make diet counseling effective at scaring off overweight people, rather than changing them.[15]

Over the years we've had a couple of overweight researchers in the Food and Brand Lab. These colleagues have always seemed to be pretty accurate at estimating the calorie content of all sorts of different foods. They were certainly no less accurate than the skinniest people in the Lab. This was just the opposite of what all the classic scientific studies report. Why?

To better understand this, I teamed up with a clever French researcher and good friend, Pierre Chandon. Together we discovered an important key to this mystery through research in an area called "psychophysics." It seems that when estimating almost anything—such as weight, height, brightness, loudness, sweetness, and so on—we consistently underestimate things as they get larger. For instance, we'll be fairly accurate at estimating the weight of a 2-pound rock but will grossly underestimate the weight of an 80-pound rock. We'll be fairly accurate in estimating the height of a 20-foot building but will grossly underestimate the height of a 200-foot building. Chandon believed that this same principle might apply to food.

To test this idea, we started in the lab and moved to fast-food restaurants. First, we recruited 40 people, some normal weight, some obese. We then bought 15 different-sized meals that ranged from 445 to 1,780 calories. We asked each person to estimate the number of calories in each of the 15 meals. The results were alike, regardless of the person's weight. The smaller the meal, the more accurate people were at estimating its calorie level. The larger the meal, the less accurate they were. Almost everyone estimated huge 1,780 calorie meals as having only 1,000 calories or so. There were no differences in the estimates of the skinniest people or the largest people.

At high levels, all of us—normal weight and overweight alike—underestimate calorie levels with mathematical predictability.[16]

We confirmed our findings when we ran a "real world" study at a number of fast-food restaurants. As people finished lunch, we asked 139 of them what they had ordered and how many calories they thought they ate (and drank). The more people had eaten, the less accurate they were. Someone eating a small, 300-calorie hamburger and a salad would underestimate the calories by about 10 percent, but someone eating a 900-calorie monsterburger would underestimate it by a whopping 40 percent. It didn't matter whether the person was skinny or huge, male or female— the bigger the meal, the less they thought they ate.

It is "meal size," not "people size," that determines how accurate we'll be at estimating how many calories we've eaten.[17] That Popsicle-stick skinny person eating a 2,000-calorie Thanksgiving dinner will underestimate how much he's eaten by just as much as the heavy person eating a 2,000-calorie pizza dinner. The trouble is that the heavy person tends to eat a whole lot more large meals.

Reengineering Strategy #2: See All You Eat

Our eyes are *not* typically bigger than our stomach. In fact, they're often better than our stomach at telling us when we're full. For instance, the Super Bowl partiers eyed their chicken bones to tell them when they'd eaten enough. As long as we help out our eyes (and don't trick them with refillable soup bowls), they can help us reengineer our food life.

- **See it *before* you eat it.** We find that when people preplate their food, they eat about 14 percent less than when they take smaller amounts and go back for seconds or thirds. Put everything you want to eat on a plate *before* you start eating—snacks, dinners, ice cream, and even chips. Your stomach won't have to count and you won't have to remember how much you took. Instead of eating directly out of a package or box, put your snack in a separate dish and leave the box in the kitchen. You'll be less likely to eat more, and more, and more.
- **See it *while* you eat it.** When you're eating chicken wings or ribs, you'll eat less if you see what you've already eaten. The same is true with beverages—it's easy to forget how much soda you've had if there's nothing to remind you. One way is to count beverage empties. For instance, if you want to keep friends from overimbibing at your next dinner party, keep the empty wine bottles on the table and pour refills into fresh glasses, without clearing the others. This should help stretch your supply of North Dakota wine.

3

Surveying the Tablescape

FLIP THROUGH YOUR RECENT memories and find a visual snapshot of a typical dinner at home. Visualize the tablescape—the placement and the types of dishes, silverware, drinking glasses, and serving bowls. Picture where the food was located on table, how it was arranged, and how much variety there was at that meal. If you can, recall where the food was stored before it was prepared and what its packaging looked like.

Maybe you can visualize this; but probably you can't. After all, the tablescape of a meal seems like a meaningless detail in the daily drama of our lives. Most of us are more concerned about our frustrations at work, our son's grades, and our undone to-do list than we are about dinner-table details.

And yet the tablescape you were asked to visualize is filled with hidden persuaders. Each of the innocuous-looking items on the table—packages, dishes, glasses, and the variety of foods—can increase how much we eat by well over 20 percent. They can also be used to decrease how much we eat. Either way—up or down—the impact they have on us will be mindless.

King-Size Packages and
the Power of Norms

Americans are often shocked when they check out the typical kitchen in Europe or in Asia. Where is the island in the middle, where are the rows of cabinets, the pantry, the refrigerator the size of a Suburu? The micro-size of most foreign kitchens and refrigerators would render an American home nearly unsellable.

The danger of our huge American kitchens is that they give us lots of space to fill up with huge American packages. We can buy bigger boxes of pasta, restaurant-size jars of spaghetti sauce, and chunkier packages of ground beef. Some of us even buy an extra refrigerator or deep freezer.

These bigger packages can save us money and save us an extra trip to the supermarket because we ran out of something. They also lead us to make bigger meals and eat more food.

Imagine that a professor from a local university approaches an organization to which you belong—such as a Parent Teacher Association—and proposes a fund-raiser for your organization. He'll donate $20 to your organization in your name if you come to the school kitchen one evening and make a spaghetti dinner for yourself and your spouse. He'll even provide the food—a medium-size box of spaghetti, a medium-size jar of spaghetti sauce, and one pound of ground beef.

What you won't know, however, is that half of the people in your organization will receive not the medium size, but a large box of spaghetti, a large jar of spaghetti sauce, and two pounds of ground beef. What you also won't know is that after you finish dinner, he'll weigh how much spaghetti, pasta, and ground beef you have left, and how much you cooked but didn't eat.

We've done dozens of similar studies with dozens of different foods. With spaghetti, for instance, we found that the people who were given the large package of pasta, sauce, and meat typically prepared 23 percent more—around 150 extra calories—than those given the medium packages.

Did they eat it all? Yes. We find over and over that if people serve themselves, they tend to eat most—92 percent—of what they serve.[1] For many of the breakfast, lunch, and dinner foods we have studied, the result is about the same— people eat 20–25 percent more on average from the larger packages.[2] For snack foods, it's even worse.

On another occasion we asked 40 adults at a PTA meeting to watch a videotape and provide some feedback about it. As a thank you, they were *each* given a bag of M&M's— either a half-pound bag or a one-pound bag—to enjoy while they watched the tape. In reality, we didn't really care what they thought about the tape, we only cared how many M&M's they ate while watching it. After they finished the video, we weighed the remains in their M&M's bag.

The results were dramatic. Those who were given a half-pound bag ate an average of 71 M&M's. Those who were given the one-pound bag ate an average of 137 M&M's, almost twice as many—264 calories more. Sure, a person saves some money by buying the big bag, but if he decides to watch a hundred videos in the next year, it will also cost him nine pounds of extra weight.[3]

The bottom line: We all consume more from big packages,

whatever the product. Give people
a large bag of dog food, they pour
more. Give them a large bottle of
liquid plant food, they pour more.
Give them a large shampoo
bottle or container of laun-
dry detergent, they pour
more. In fact, with the 47
products we've examined, the
bigger the package, the more
they use. There was only one
exception: liquid bleach.
Most people know that if
they use too much, their
socks and shirts experience a religious conversion. They become holy.

Why do we automatically eat (or pour) more from big
packages? Because big packages (like big portions) suggest
a consumption norm—what is appropriate or normal to use
or eat.[4]

As all of our studies suggest, we can eat about 20 percent more or 20 percent less without really being aware of
it. Because of this, we look for cues and signals that tell us
how much to eat. One of these signals is the size of the package. When we bring a big package into our kitchen, we think
it's typical, normal, and appropriate to mix and to serve
more than if the package were smaller.

Although we may not finish the two-pound box of spaghetti when we make dinner for two, it makes us think it's
normal to take a few more bites than we would if it were a

one-pound box. It bumps up our consumption norms and leads us to bump up how much we serve ourselves.[5]

Drinking Glass Illusions

Big packages have plenty of kitchen accomplices. It's been estimated that 72 percent of our calories come from food that we eat from bowls, plates, and glasses.[6] These containers can create persuasive visual illusions that cause us to misjudge the amount of food they contain.

Who cares? Dieters care, athletes care, and bartenders care. For instance, if we give you a tall, skinny glass and a short, wide glass, you'll drink 25–30 percent more out of one than the other. Which one should you choose?

You may remember the Horizontal-Vertical illusion from a brain-teasers book you had as a kid. This common illusion looks like an upside-down capital "T." The horizontal and vertical lines are exactly the same length, but virtually everyone thinks the vertical line is longer: 18 to 20 percent longer, on average.

The Horizontal-Vertical Illusion:
Which Line Is Longer?

Our brains have a basic tendency to overfocus on the height of objects at the expense of their width. Take the Gateway Arch in St. Louis. Commemorating the Louisiana Purchase, it's a remarkable sight that greets anyone crossing the Mississippi River from Illinois into St. Louis.

The arch is America's tallest man-made monument. It is also exactly the same height as width—630 feet tall and 630 feet wide. Despite this, none of the 11,000 tourists who visit the arch on an average day says, "Wow . . . look how wide it is." No way, we all stare at the height.

What does all this have to do with drinking glasses?

To find out, let's visit a health and nutrition camp— the kind of camp where teenagers and preteens go for the summer to lose a few pounds and to detox from years of a Cheetos-based diet. There they learn how to estimate portion size, count calories, eat better, and exercise. These camps tend to be expensive—$7,500 for the whole summer.[7] If a camper loses only three pounds during his stay, it costs his parents $2,500 a pound. As a result, the kids are motivated to lose weight, they learn how to lose weight, and they vigilantly avoid the things that get in the way. If anyone is resistant to visual illusions, these campers should be the ones.

To examine this, we persuaded a health and nutrition camp in New England to make a small adjustment to the cafeteria line. As the teenagers came into the dining hall one day, they were randomly given either a tall, skinny glass or a short, wide glass with the same capacity. The kids picked up their trays, went through the line as usual, took whatever food they wanted, and poured whatever drink they wanted. At the other end of the line, the kids were surprised to be greeted by one of the researchers, who asked them to estimate how much they had poured, and who weighed their glasses to see how accurate they were.

The campers who'd been given the tall, thin glasses poured about 5.5 ounces. But for those campers given the short, wide glasses, it was a different story. They poured an average of 9.6 ounces—74 percent more than their tall-glass buddies. The real surprise: They estimated that they had poured only 7 ounces.

Adults don't do much better. Koert van Ittersum and I repeated this study with musicians at a jazz improvisation camp in Western Massachusetts. On two consecutive mornings, these jazz musicians, who were on average 37 years old, were offered breakfast accompanied by a tall or short glass. Even though they were older and wiser, they still got fatter if they used the short glasses. The people given a short, wide glass poured an average of 19 percent more juice or soft drink than those given the tall, thin glass.[8]

Not convinced? Remember, the real danger of these kitchen traps is that almost every single person in the world believes they're immune to them. They might say, "Sure, this works with clueless teenagers and for jazz musicians with the munchies, but it would never work on me."

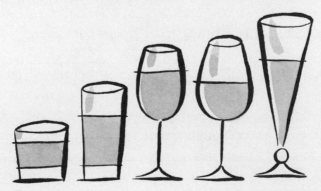

Okay, but let's suppose we could find professional pourers. Suppose we could find experts who are paid to pour the exact same amount of liquid—1.5 ounces, one "shot"—into thousands of glasses a year. They have poured this amount over and over again. Surely they wouldn't be fooled by the shape of a glass.

These experts are easy to find. They're called bartenders. For this experiment, we recruited 45 professional bartenders in Philadelphia:[9] men and women, young and old, tiny and tattooed. Some were pouring Dom Pérignon for $150 lunches in Center City; others were pouring unbranded shots for Dollar Tequila Night in West Philly.

We went into their own bars, so everything would feel natural to them, and we asked them to pour rum for a rum and coke, gin for a gin and tonic, whiskey for a whiskey on the rocks, and vodka for a vodka tonic. They knew how much they were supposed to pour. In all cases, it was one shot, 1.5 ounces.

The catch: They couldn't use their "one-Mississippi, two-Mississippi" pour spouts, and they couldn't use a measuring cup or shot glass. They had to pour the old-fashioned way, straight out of the bottle. We then gave them either a tall, skinny, 11-ounce highball glass, or a short, fat, 11-ounce tumbler. These were veteran bartenders, with over five years of experience each.

What happened? Those who were given the tall, skinny glasses were almost exactly on target. They poured 1.6 ounces. Those who had been given the short, fat glasses were a different story. Even though they had poured drinks for over five years, and even though they always poured the same amount, they poured an average of 2.1 ounces: 37 percent more than their target. We even asked an additional 41 bartenders to "Please take your time when pouring." They still overpoured. So much for experience.[10]

The Horizontal-Vertical illusion makes a difference.[11] While it may not matter if you're drinking water, it does matter if you're pouring more calories of a soft drink than you intended.[12] And it really, really matters if someone ends up pouring—and drinking—more alcohol than they intended. A lot of people may have to pay for that mistake. It's one thing to say to yourself, "I will not overpour into this wide glass," but if bartenders can't even avoid doing so, what hope do the rest of us have? It's a lot easier to simply say, "Let's only use the tall, skinny glasses." After seeing that even expert pourers get fooled, most of us from the Lab replaced the short, wide juice glasses in our kitchens and kept the taller ones. One of our researchers even replaced his large, wide red-wine glasses with smaller, slender glasses intended for white wine.

Big Plates, Big Spoons, Big Servings

Here's another visual illusion you might remember from those brain-teaser books of your youth: the Size-Contrast illusion. This involves a medium-size dot surrounded by small circles and a second medium-size dot surrounded by much larger circles. The second dot appears much smaller than the first, even though it's exactly the same size (and even if you know the trick). Essentially, we use background objects as a benchmark for estimating size. For instance, if we see a photo of a six-foot man standing next to a tricycle, we think he is taller than if he were shown next to a cement truck.

The Size-Contrast Illusion: Which Black Dot Is Bigger?

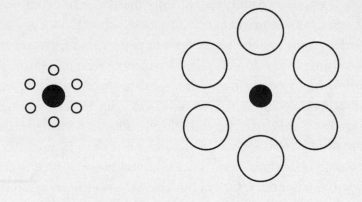

Now translate this to the tablescape. If you spoon four ounces of mashed potatoes onto a 12-inch plate, it will look like a lot less than if you had spooned it onto an 8-inch plate. Even if you intended to limit your portion size, the larger plate would likely influence you to serve more. And since we all tend to finish what we serve ourselves, we would probably end up eating it all.

Again, even professionals are fooled by this illusion. In 2001, the TV show *20/20* visited our Lab to film some of our research. To celebrate what was supposed to be the end of the filming—the "wrap party"—there was an ice-cream social. All of the distinguished professors from the Nutritional

Science Division and all of the hardworking Ph.D. students were invited to share in the celebration.

But the filming was not really over, and the ice-cream social was actually an experiment. When our guests showed up, they were given either medium-size 17-ounce bowls or large-size 34-ounce bowls; then they were invited to go through the line and take as much of four different kinds of ice cream as they wanted. We also varied the size of the scoops that we put in the ice cream. Some held two ounces, some three ounces. When people reached the end of the line, one of the experimenters handed them a survey while they weighed their bowl of ice cream. All the while, the cameras were rolling.

Surely our guests wouldn't be affected by something as mundane as the size of the bowls and scoops? They think, sleep, lecture, study, and eat nutrition. They've written hundreds of top-level research papers on nutrition.

None of that mattered. Those who were given the huge bowls dished out huge amounts. In fact, they dished about 31 percent more—127 more calories' worth of ice cream. It only makes things worse if you give them a big scoop. People with a large bowl and a three-ounce scoop dished out 57 percent more ice cream than those given a smaller bowl and smaller scoop.[13]

Big dishes and big spoons are big trouble. As the size of our dishes increases, so does the amount we scoop onto them.

They cause us to serve ourselves more because they make the food look so small. If you take a medium-size hamburger and serve it to a person on a saucer, they estimate it as having 18 percent more calories than if you serve it to them on a normal-size plate. The same thing is true with desserts. When presented on a large plate, people underestimate the number of calories in a piece of pie or cake compared to when it's presented to them on a smaller plate.

Serving-size norms were different 50 years ago. How do we know this? One way is by comparing Grandmother's 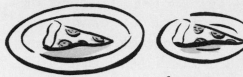 dinner plates with our own. An antiques dealer told me that when people shopping for antique plates find a pattern they like, they often take a dinner plate up to him and say, "I like these cute little salad plates. Do you have matching dinner plates?" One woman even asked if he had any duplicates of the serving platters that she could use as dinner plates.

The Super Bowl Intelligentsia

This bowl bias seems straightforward, and the solution seems simple. Tell people about their bias, and the problem will be solved.

In the spring of 2003 I gave a research presentation about size cues to the National Academy of Science in Washington, D.C. One of the scientists in the audience mused that these cues must disproportionately hurt the less-educated, because "Surely the size of serving bowls, scoops, and plates couldn't possibly influence how much an intelligent, informed person eats."

Let's see.

We'll take 63 sharp, competitive graduate students at a top research university. We'll devote a full 90-minute class session just before Christmas vacation to talking about the size bias. We'll lecture to them, show them videos, have them go through a demonstration, and even break them into small groups to discuss how people could prevent themselves from "being tricked" by bigger serving bowls. We'll use just about every educational method short of doing an interpretive dance. At the end of the 90 minutes, they will be sick of the topic, sick of the professor, and sick of school.[14] Why? Because this is obvious and because they're intelligent and informed.

Six weeks later, we'll see what they remember.

In late January, we invited these students to a Super Bowl party at a sports bar, and 40 accepted. When they arrived, they were led to one of two rooms to get their snacks for the game. Those who were led to the first room found a table with two huge gallon bowls of Chex Mix. They were given a plate and asked to take as much as they wanted. As they got to the end of the line, we asked them to fill out a brief survey about Super Bowl commercials.

There was only one empty corner of the table where they could put their plate while filling out the survey. What they didn't know was that there was a scale under the tablecloth and that the amount they had served themselves was being weighed and recorded.

In the second room, everything was the same except that the Chex Mix had been put out in four half-gallon bowls.

What did our size-bias experts do? The students who served themselves from the gallon bowls took 53 percent more Chex Mix than those serving themselves from half-gallon bowls. An hour later we cleared away their plates, which had identification codes on the bottom. Not only did those who served themselves from the large bowls take 53 percent more, they also ate more (59 percent more).[15]

No one is immune to serving-size norms—not even "intelligent, informed" people who have been lectured on the subject *ad nauseam*.

In the end, setting the table with the wrong dinner plates or serving bowls—the big ones—sets the stage for overeating. And there are heavyweight consequences, especially when you're sitting in front of a wide variety of food.

The Temptation of Variety

Atkins-mania and the low-carb diet. For a while, it was the rage. Nearly everyone was on the low-carb bandwagon or had friends who had experienced miraculous results. A woman in one low-carb ad even claimed the diet had changed her from a "circus act to a supermodel." The basic deal was "Eat anything you want and as much as you want as long as it doesn't have refined carbohydrates." No bread, rice, pasta, potatoes, or sugar, but all the beef, butter, and cheesy broccoli you can stand.

The Atkins Diet worked initially because it made dieting a mindless activity. There were bad guys (carbohydrates) and good guys (meat and vegetables), and very little variety.

The good news: The Atkins Diet worked. The bad news: It was boring to eat just meat and vegetables.

Capitalism came to the rescue. Nearly every red-blooded American food company tried to remedy the boredom by giving us more options. They gave us low-carb cereals, desserts, and beers. Russell Stover even gave us low-carb chocolate and caramel turtles. At the diet's highest (or perhaps lowest) point, Christopher Atkins, who was Brooke Shields' co-star in the 1980 movie *The Blue Lagoon,* came out with the Atkins Cookie, apparently riding the coincidence of his last name.

Atkins lost its magic. In the old days, there were only meat and vegetables. Now there were hundreds and hundreds of "low carb" nonmeat and nonvegetable foods. And instead of happy, svelte, protein lovers who had dropped 40 pounds, the low-carb diet began to produce continuous snackers who were mystified that they only lost 4 pounds. Although everything they ate was according to the letter of the Atkins law, they were eating too much of it.

There have always been food-restriction diets, ranging from the Grapefruit Diet to the Cabbage Soup Diet. They all have two things in common: 1) You can only eat a limited variety of foods, but 2) you can eat an unlimited amount of them. They all work to some extent because people get sick and tired of eating the same foods. As a result, they eventually start eating less. It's like going to a buffet that has all the roast beef you can eat. You'll never eat as much as you will at the buffet with 60 different types of foods.

Increasing the variety of a food increases how much everyone eats. To demonstrate this, Dr. Barbara Rolls' team at Penn State has showed that if people are offered an assortment with three different flavors of yogurt, they're likely to consume an average of 23 percent more than if offered only one flavor.[16]

This behavior results from what is called "sensory specific

satiety." In other words, our senses get numbed or sated if they continually experience the same stimulus.[17]

An extreme example involves people who work in packing plants (less euphemistically known as slaughterhouses). These folks are not greeted with a spring-fresh odor when they arrive at work every day. The odor in a packing plant is so horrible, your eyes will water. Fortunately, after a while, you stop noticing it. That is why, by lunchtime, the workers can eat their ham and cheese sandwiches and smell nothing but the Velveeta. Although their ability to smell the packing plant has "burned out," they are still able to smell other things.[18]

Sensory specific satiety also affects our taste buds. The first bite of anything is almost always the best. The second a little less, the third less again. At some point, we're tired of the yogurt or cake. But if we add two more types of yogurt, or if we add ice cream to the cake, our taste buds are back to the races.

This is why we eat more when there is variety. It's a simple idea, but it has a lot of implications. If you're trying to control your weight, one obvious implication is not to eat every meal at the Kung Pao Garden's 2,000-item buffet. You can also stop thinking that every meal should consist of four or five different foods. And what about the reception or party where you're tempted with dozens of merciless morsels? A smart strategy is never to have more than two items on your plate at any one time. You can go back if you're still hungry, but the lack of variety slows you down, and you end up eating less.

There's something strange about the variety effect, however. As my colleague Barbara Kahn and I discovered, it's not entirely a matter of sensory specific satiety. We not only eat more when there is more variety, we also eat more if we simply *think* there is more. That is, if our eyes lead us to believe we have more choices, we serve ourselves more, and we dutifully clean our plates.

We tested this on international students who were beginning an MBA program. As part of their weeklong orientation, the students were invited to attend the movie *Pearl Harbor* and receive free popcorn, soft drinks, and candy. The candy was jelly beans, and they were presented in one of two ways. Half of the moviegoers were offered jelly beans in a tray that was divided into six parts, each of which was filled with 200 jelly beans of the same kind. One part was filled with cherry jelly beans, one with lime jelly beans, one with orange, and so on.[19]

The other half of the moviegoers were offered the same six flavors of jelly beans, but instead of being neatly organized by color, they were all mixed together. Who do you think took more, the person eating from the organized tray or the person eating from the disorganized tray? The grad students faced with the organized tray took about 12 jelly beans and headed off to enjoy the movie. But those people presented with the disorganized assortment took an average of 23 jelly beans, nearly twice as many. In both cases, the number and flavors of jelly beans are identical, yet mixing them up nearly doubles how many a person takes and eats.[20]

What about colors? What if we do not change the taste of foods, but only change their color? For instance, what would happen if we gave two people huge bowls of M&M's to snack on while they watched a video? The only difference between the bowls is that one has 7 colors of M&M's and the other has 10 colors.[21] Most people know that all M&M's taste alike. The color is just added to the coating. There's no way they should eat different amounts.

But they do. The person with 10 colors will eat 43 more M&M's (99 versus 56) than his friend with 7 colors. He does so because he thinks there's more variety, which increases how much he thinks he'll like the M&M's and how much he thinks is normal to eat.

A common practice at parties is to take a limited number of snacks or hors d'oeuvres and put them on smaller trays and spread them around the room. Starving graduate-student hosts have perfected this to an art form.

Instead of having three really large bowls of chips, peanuts, and candy, these shrewd, cost-conscious hosts and hostesses might put the chips in four small bowls, the peanuts in four small bowls, and the candy in four small bowls. It makes people think there's a lot more food—and a lot more variety. Exact same variety, but very different perceptions.

Two MBA-student holiday parties at my house seemed to be the perfect time for a demonstration to prospective Lab members. One Tuesday night, one-gallon bowls of each of the three different snacks were set out on the red-and-green-decorated dining room table. We counted how many people were at the party and weighed the snacks that remained at the end. The next day we e-mailed the people and asked them to rate how much snack variety there was the night before on a 1–9 scale (little variety–much variety). The following week I had another party, where each of the three snacks was split into four one-quart bowls.

At which party is the average person likely to eat more—

the 12-bowl party or the 3-bowl party? Even though the amount of food was the same, putting the food in 12 bowls increased how much people ate by 18 percent. When we asked our guests to rate the variety, sure enough, they gave higher scores to the party with the 12 bowls.[22]

Reengineering Strategy #3: Be Your Own Tablescaper

You can control your tablescape, or your tablescape will control you. When we modify the tablescape in our Lab, we can easily cut down how much a person eats by 15 percent or more. Here's where you can start:

- **Mini-size your boxes and bowls.** The bigger the package you pour from—be it cereal boxes on the table or spaghetti in the kitchen—the more you will eat: 20 to 30 percent more for most foods. How can you get your supersized savings and still eat less? Repackage your jumbo box into smaller Ziploc bags or Tupperware containers, and serve it up in smaller dishes. The smaller the box, the less you make, and the less you eat. The smaller the serving dish, the less you take, and the less you eat.
- **Become an illusionist.** Six ounces of goulash on an 8-inch plate is a nice-size serving. Six ounces on a 12-inch plate looks like a tiny appetizer. Make visual illusions work for you. After you drop your platter-size dinner plates off at Goodwill, pick up a nice set of mid-size plates that you can be proud of.

With glasses, think slender if you want to be slender. If you don't fill your glass, you'll tend to pour 30 percent more into a wide glass than into a tall, slender one. It's easier to get rid of your wide glasses than to consistently remind yourself not to use them.

- **Beware of the double danger of leftovers.** The more side dishes and little bowls of leftovers you bring out of the refrigerator, the more you will eat. If you're bringing out carrot sticks, this probably doesn't matter—but are you? The second danger of leftovers? They signal that you made too much— and probably ate too much—of the original meal.

Got healthy food on your mind? You can throw the switch on these three tips and it will encourage the gang to eat more than they otherwise would.

4

The Hidden
Persuaders Around Us

O N A N Y G I V E N D A Y of the week you can log on to
eBay.com and bid on a talking candy dish. These dishes
come in all shapes, but the most popular one is a pink pig
with a hollowed-out back where you can pile the candy.
This is no run-of-the-mill pig dish. This one contains a sen-
sor that detects when your hand is reaching into it. It re-
sponds with an unmistakable, continuous, "oink, oink, oink,
oink" until you either abandon your candy quest or defi-
antly snatch one and retreat to a corner to feast in quiet.

There are only a couple of oink dishes up for bid on eBay
on any given day, and they usually sell for around $12.
Given this low price point, we're probably not going to see
a herd of spin-offs that include the Oink Refrigerator, the
Oink Cupboard, and the Oink Office Desk. That's too bad
for us mindless eaters. These are all places that are booby-
trapped with hidden persuaders that can make us overeat.

The "See-Food" Trap

There was a silly one-liner that was a big hit in my fourth grade hot-lunch room for about two weeks. After someone ravenously finished a large lunch, a kid would say, "You must be on the See-Food Diet—because you eat everything you see."

Most people are on see-food diets to some degree. Simply seeing (or smelling) a food can lead us to want to devour it. Think you have the willpower to avoid that little dish of chocolates you have sitting on your office desk or in your living room? Think again.

Suppose we give an office building full of secretaries nice covered dishes of 30 Hershey's Kisses as a personal, not-to-be-shared gift for Secretary's Week. The glass dishes are identical except for one detail: Half are clear and half are white so that they totally hide the chocolates if the lid is on. Now suppose that every night after the secretaries go home we count how many they have eaten, refill the dish, and continue this for two weeks.

Dr. Jim Painter and I did this study and had fun doing it—everybody loves free chocolates. Unfortunately, the results aren't so fun for anyone who's trying to watch what they eat.[1]

Secretaries who had been given candies in clear desktop dishes were caught

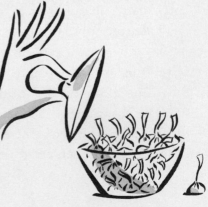

with their hand in the candy dish 71 percent more often (7.7 versus 4.6 times) as those given white dishes. Every day that dish was on their desk they ate 77 more calories. Over a year, that candy dish would have added over five pounds of extra weight. What is a little bit scary is that none of them would have probably known where those pounds came from.

It's not just candy on the desk. This same principle of visibility can follow us through the day. In a classic line of studies started at Columbia University in the 1960s, researchers put a plate of food (such as small chicken salad sandwiches) in front of people during lunch. Some would be given food covered with transparent wrap and others were given food covered with aluminum foil. In nearly all these studies, people ate more of the food in transparent wrap than in aluminum foil.[2]

Why does this happen? We eat more of these visible "see-foods" because we think about them more. Every time we see the candy jar we have to decide whether we want a Hershey's Kiss or whether we don't. Every time we see it, we have to say no to something that is tasty and tempting. If we see that temptress of a candy jar every five minutes, it means needing to say no 12 times the first hour, 12 times the second hour, and so on. Eventually some of those no's turn into yes's. Usually in the form of "Well, okay, just this once . . ."

Out of sight, out of mind. In sight, in mind.

Interestingly, however, there's a more subtle and hidden reason why the siren song of the candy dish and the cookie jar traps us. Simply thinking of food can make you hungry.[3] Just like Pavlov's dogs, we salivate (subtly) when we hear, see, or smell something we associate with food—like a shiny foil-wrapped piece of milk chocolate. Even though we haven't touched the chocolate, our pancreas may begin to secrete insulin, a chemical used to metabolize the upcoming sugar rush we're planning. This insulin lowers our blood sugar level, which makes us feel hungry. While drooling has never hurt anyone, the more actively you salivate, the more likely you are to be impulsive and to overeat. Studies have even shown that the more we like the food the faster we'll chew and swallow it.[4]

But we don't need to have candy in front of us for it to be on the top of our mind. All we have to do is visualize it. Simply thinking about food—thinking about whether we should go the mail room for a stale donut, or thinking we should take a break to walk down to the candy machine "just to see what's there"—has the same effect.

Take two guys in side-by-side cubicles—Will and George—and two dozen stale donuts in the mail room. George saw the donuts when he first got to work and has been thinking about them all morning. Every five minutes he thinks of them, and every five minutes he says no. Eventually, however, the no's are more difficult, so he gets up from his desk to go get a donut. Will, on the other hand, doesn't know the donuts are there, but he decides to go down and pick up his mail. Both arrive there at the same time. Who will eat more?

Smart money would bet on George. George's eating is premeditated, Will's is more impulsive. The beauty of impulse eating may be that you end up eating less—when you do eat—than someone who has been thinking about the food for hours. The more you think of something, the more of it you'll eat.[5]

The "Hide the See-Food" Diet

Out of sight is out of mind. If the candy dish sits on your desk, you consistently have to make a heroic decision whether you will resist the chocolate that has been giving you the eye all day. The easy solution is to lose the dish, move the dish, or replace the candy with something you personally don't like. Same thing with the cookie jar. It can either make a debut at a local yard sale, or the cookies can be replaced with fruit.

You can also make the see-food diet work for you. Make healthy foods easy to see, and less healthy foods hard to see. Fruit bowls can replace cookie jars. Healthy foods can migrate to the front, eye-level shelves of the refrigerator.

But all is not lost, because the see-food diet also works with the good stuff. Rohit Deshpandé and I tested this idea during the spring thaw after a long New Hampshire winter when I was a professor at Dartmouth.

Soup is a reasonably healthy food, and we wanted to see if making it really, really vivid to a person would make them more likely to eat it in the upcoming weeks. (Psychologists call this "priming.") So we asked 93 people to write down a detailed description of the most recent time they ate soup—what had happened earlier that day, what type of soup they had, what they ate with it, how it tasted, how it made them feel when they were eating it, and what they thought of the meal after they finished. This was about a full page of writing about soup. Another 94 people were simply asked to write down their most recent experience with an unrelated product.

The results were dramatic. At the end of the study, the people who had thought about the last time they had eaten soup anticipated they would eat more than twice as much soup in the next month as the non-primed group told us.

What about the visual temptations that we can't control . . . the convenience stores and fast-food places?

A roommate of mine who had a weakness for Slurpees found himself stopping at a certain 7-Eleven convenience store each afternoon. He just couldn't help himself. If he slowed down at the corner stoplight, he said, his car became possessed and turned into the 7-Eleven parking lot. As time passed and his clothes started becoming tight, he decided that if he couldn't keep his car from driving into 7-Eleven, he would take a different route home, zigzagging around the temptation. If the siren song of 7-Eleven or of Dunkin' Donuts is too difficult to resist, there are two choices: Lash yourself to the steering wheel, or don't drive by them.

In his book *The Ultimate Weight Solution,* Dr. Phil McGraw describes the siren song of his own kitchen.[6]

I am invariably hungry when I come home at the end of the day. For the longest time, I would enter the house through a door that led me through the kitchen. I would tell myself repeatedly that I was not going to snack before dinner. Sometimes the emotion of willpower would carry me, sometimes it would not. As I cruised through the kitchen, the environment was full of temptation, and I'd start grabbing junk foods, right and left. Maybe they were cookies on a platter one day, a chocolate cake the next, or some other food I would quickly consume. It was not unusual for me to wolf down anywhere between 1,500 and 10,000 calories in one sitting ("standing" would be a more apt description), shower, then sit down for a full dinner.

The solution? He changed his route and came in the front door instead of the back door. Others have used the police crime-scene strategy and put up "DO NOT ENTER" masking tape across the kitchen doorways between meals, but this would be too extreme for most of us. There are two basic tactics for avoiding the temptation of the see-food diet: 1) Move visible food, and 2) if it can't be moved, move around it.

Convenience:
Would You Walk a Mile for a Caramel?

One of the most famous books on food psychology also has one of the most infamous, cringingly politically incorrect titles ever published. *Obese Humans and Rats* was written by the late, great Columbia University professor Stanley Schachter and a team of clever researchers that included Judith Rodin, C. Peter Herman, and Patti Pliner.[7] It distilled thousands of person-hours' (and rat-hours') worth of research to show that many of the same factors that make rats fat can make humans fat.

If the book had to be summed up in one sentence, it

would be this: The more hassle it is to eat, the less we eat. If white rats in cages have to press a little food lever 10 times before they are rewarded with food pellets, they eat often. If they have to press it 100 times, they make do with less.

It's the same with us. If we had to press little levers 100 times before we were given a cupcake, we wouldn't eat as much either. If we had to run through a long maze before we got our pint of chocolate chip cookie dough ice cream, we would usually decide it wasn't worth it.

Inconvenient foods that take a lot of effort to obtain and prepare seem to have an even greater influence on people who are obese.[8] In one study, Schachter's team invited people into their office to be enrolled in a study. As soon as the person arrived, the researcher would pretend to be called away. On the way out the door he would say, "I've got to take care of something real quick. There are some almonds here on my desk. Have a seat and help yourself. I'll be back in 15 minutes." Half the time, the almonds on the desk were shelled; half the time they were unshelled.

When the researcher left, people of normal weight would generally eat one or two almonds whether or not they were shelled. This was not the case with obese people. They tended to eat the almonds only if they were already shelled and didn't involve any work. If the almonds were still in the shell, the obese people tended to leave them alone.

Even though we all let our environment tell us when and how much we should eat, some people are more influenced by it than others. But no one is exempt from the power of convenience. Let us take a look at desk-bound secretaries again.

Remember how we celebrated Secretary's Week—with candy dishes full of 30 Hershey's Kisses for their desks? Jim Painter and I did something similar with another group of secretaries. Except this time we gave everyone clear, lidded candy dishes that we rotated among three locations in their office. During the first week a secretary would find that her candy dish was on the corner of her desk. The next week, it would be in the top left-hand desk drawer. The last week, it would be on a file cabinet six feet from her desk. Other secretaries would be given their chocolates in a different order, but the three places were always the same—on the desk, in the desk, and six feet from the desk.[9]

By now you can predict what happened. The typical secretary ate about nine chocolates a day if they were sitting on her desk staring right at her. That's about 225 extra calories a day. If she had to go to the effort of opening the desk drawer, she did so only six times a day. If she had to get up and walk six feet to get a chocolate, she ate only four. In the same way that it's not worth the effort for an Eskimo to locate and overeat mangos, it's not always worth the effort for us to walk six feet for a chocolate. The basic principle is convenience.

However, something else might be going on here, as well. When we talked to the secretaries after the study, many of them mentioned that having six feet between them and the candy gave them enough time to think twice whether they really wanted it. It gave them time to talk themselves out of having another chocolate. When a chocolate tempted them from one arm's-length away, the interval between impulse and action was too short to matter.

Let's return to Schachter's white rats. In one clever set of

Take the Chinese Buffet Chopstick Test

Eating with chopsticks can be a hassle. People eat slower and eat less per bite. This is why dieters are often told to eat with chopsticks. So who do you suppose is more likely to use a fork when eating in a Chinese restaurant—a normal-weight person or an obese person?

We decided to find out. We observed 100 normal-weight diners and 100 obese diners at Chinese buffets in California, Minnesota, and New York, and we noted whether they were eating with chopsticks or silverware.

Out of 33 people eating with chopsticks, 26 were normal weight and only 7 were obese.[10]

Take the Chinese Buffet Chopstick test. Next time you find yourself at a Chinese restaurant, check out who's eating with the chopsticks and who has a fork in their hand.

studies, researchers filled a large room with a number of gymnastic balance beams that were connected in a mazelike pattern. At the end of one balance beam was a container of tasty rat food. At the other end of a different beam was a box where a white rat was nested. Whenever the rat was hungry, he would waddle out across the balance beams, eat until full, and waddle back to his white castle. Ah, but to make it interesting, the researchers periodically filled the air with the scent of a predatory hawk. Now it was a great deal less convenient (and more risky) for the rat to go snacking whenever the urge hit, because he needed to quickly run to the food, eat it fast, and run back, all while keeping an eye on the sky. When they put the hawk scent in the air, the rat was much less likely to go get food, and when it did, it ate its meal much more quickly and consumed much less. Although we're not endangered by raptors on our way to the refrigerator, this study shows that our inborn quest for convenient food is probably there for a reason.[11]

Cafeteria studies show this in a way that does not involve rats (we hope). In a cafeteria, as in our home, the convenience of a food pretty much determines whether we will eat it or not. If people have to go to a separate lunch line to pay for candy and potato chips, they buy less.[12] If the salad bar is farther away from the table, they will eat less salad. That's not surprising.

But there's even a limit to how much work we will do for something we love as much as candy and ice cream. One cafeteria tested this by leaving the glass lid of an ice-cream cooler closed on some days and open on other days. The ice-cream cooler was in the exact same location, and people

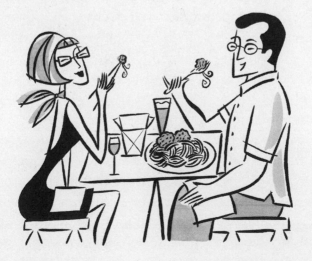

could always see the ice cream. All that varied was whether they had to go through the effort of opening the lid in order to get it. Even that was too much work for many people. If the lid was closed, only 14 percent of the diners decided it was worth the modest effort to open it. If the lid was open, 30 percent decided it was ice-cream time.[13]

If the effort of opening a lid prevents many people from eating ice cream, why don't companies make lidless ice-cream freezers? They have, and they are popular in many crowded tourist areas in Europe. The ice-cream-loving Europeans have developed freezers that cool the ice cream bars from the bottom. Because there's no lid on the freezer, there's one less barrier to grabbing, buying, and eating ice cream, and one less barrier to keep us from taking the time to decide whether we really want ice cream or not.

The power of convenience even applies to milk and water. In the military, dehydration can have deadly results. Studies are continually being done to determine how to increase fluid intake.[14] In one mess-hall study, soldiers drank almost twice as much water (81 percent more) when water pitchers were put on each dining table than when they were put on a side table. They drank 42 percent more milk when the milk machine was 12 feet away than when it was 25 feet away.

Just as a white rat might prefer a mediocre-tasting food pellet to the gourmet pellet that is a long, dangerous run away, we learn to prefer convenient microwave popcorn to less convenient but more tasty stove-top popcorn. And just as Eskimos don't eat mangos, the Incans never wrote cookbooks containing recipes for seal meat. Those foods are not around and they're too much of a hassle to obtain.

The Curse of the Warehouse Club

Who doesn't like a deal? Warehouse club stores, like Sam's Club, BJ's, Costco, and Pace, are great. For around $35 a year you can be an exclusive member of the club. It may not have the same cachet as your local Caddyshack Country Club, but the bargains are better. You may not get access to a swimming pool full of beautiful people or to a well-manicured golf course, but you can buy pretzels by the barrel and smoked salmon by the pallet. There are no golf carts, but there are those little flatbeds you can push around and load up to dangerous heights.

But there are a few hidden curses of warehouse clubs. Membership has its privileges, but think of what happens moments after a person (like me, for more than 20 years) pays $35 for their yearlong membership. The natural inclination is to run through the store like Julie Andrews running through the fields in *The Sound of Music,* buying enough stuff so that you can "recoup" the price of membership. If you can save $5 by buying the 48-pack of flavored seltzer water, all you have to do is load 7 of these 48-packs on the pushcart flatbed to break even on the membership deal.

So the first curse is to overspend, even on things we don't need. ("I don't know what this is, so I'll only buy three.") The second curse takes effect later, after we buy bulk food and return home. Most bulk foods come in large single-open containers (such as five-pound barrels of pretzels) and in large multi-pack containers (48 packets of instant oatmeal).

Consider the huge containers. From what we've learned

about consumption and container size, you know that you'll eat much more from these huge containers for the first seven days. After that you'll start slowing down because you become tired of the food. What happens next? These foods become "cabinet castaways," slowly migrating to the back of the cupboard, and eventually to the basement or storeroom, or the far corner of the refrigerator or freezer.[15] Out of sight, out of mind. Eventually, during spring refrigerator cleaning, you decide to throw out the food. The great bargain of

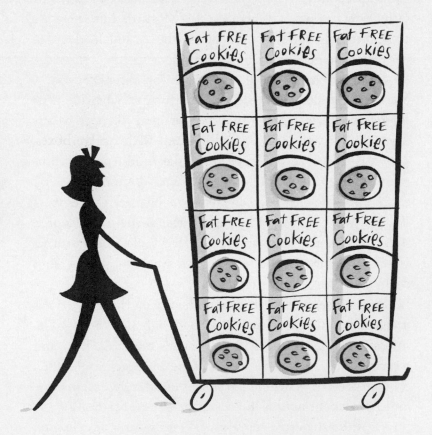

buying five pounds for $5 does not end up being so great if you eventually throw two pounds away.

Now take those multi-pack containers. Having 48 packages of almost anything in your house affects consumption in two ways. The first is what we call "the salience principle"—these 48 packages tend to get in the way. You seem to see them everywhere, they fall out of the cupboard when you open it, they pile up on the counter, and they hide other foods. As a result of their salience, you end up eating them much more frequently than you normally would, particularly if the food is convenient to eat. There they are . . . every time you want a snack.

The second reason we eat these foods so fast brings us back to the idea of "norms." Suppose you usually have two or three boxes of breakfast cereal in your cupboard. If you find yourself with only one box, it's a signal you need to buy more. But if one day you find yourself with twelve boxes, you will tend to eat them up so the "right" number will be in your cupboard, and so you'll have room for other foods.

A series of studies I conducted with marketing professor Pierre Chandon showed that the warehouse club curse mainly occurs in the first week after shopping there. We recruited warehouse club members in New Hampshire and gave them shopping baskets full of free foods, some which were in larger quantities and some in smaller quantities. These included cookies, crackers, candy, juice, ramen noodles, and microwave popcorn. We then tracked how quickly the club members consumed these foods over the next two weeks.[16]

For the first week, people ate these stockpiled foods at almost twice the normal rate. But by the end of the first week, they had started to burn out and were no longer eating

Get a Better Deal from Your Wholesale Club

- Repackage jumbo sizes into smaller bags and Tupperware containers.
- Hide the extras. If you buy 144 packs of microwave popcorn, put a few in your cupboard and pack the rest away—far away, in the basement or the very back of a closet. Make them inconvenient to track down and use.
- Reseal packages. Using tape to close a bag of chips is more of a deterrent to an impulse splurge than an easy-to-open clip.

them as frequently. After that period, the food was either gone, they were tired of it, or they threw it out because it was stale.

Are wholesale clubs a good deal when it comes to food? You certainly save money at the cash register, but you lose much of that money if you end up overbuying and having to throw food out. You also don't benefit if you end up eating the food after it stops tasting good only because you want to—ugh—"finish it up." Last, you can end up gaining weight by eating a food that you don't even like. That is the ultimate curse.

Reengineering Strategy #4:
Make Overeating a Hassle, Not a Habit

Remember what happened to the secretaries once we moved the candy dish six feet away from the desk? They ate half as many. It was a little more of a hassle to get them, and that six-foot barrier gave them the chance to rethink whether they really wanted a chocolate. It gave them a pause point. Here are some tips to give you a chance to pause:

- **Leave serving dishes in the kitchen or on a sideboard.** Like the secretaries who snatched candies and ate them before they realized it, we do the same thing with serving bowls that are right in front of us. Having them at least six feet away gives us a chance to ask if we're really that hungry. Turn this around for salad and veggies. Make sure they're firmly planted in the "pick me" spot in the middle of the table.
- **"De-convenience" tempting foods.** Take those temptresses down to a remote corner of the basement or put them in a hard-to-reach cupboard. Reseal packages and wrap the most tempting leftovers in aluminum foil and put them in the back of the refrigerator or freezer.
- **Snack only at the table and on a clean plate.** This makes it less convenient to serve, eat, and clean up after an impulse snack.

Of course, a better idea yet is to not bring impulse foods in the house to begin with. Eat before you shop, use a list, and stick to the perimeter of the store. That's where the fresh foods hang out.

5

Mindless Eating Scripts

WHEN JOHN DRAGS IN from work, he puts his things away, walks into the kitchen, looks for a snack, and starts to eat it on the way to the television. If you were to ask him why, he'd hesitate then say, "Because it's what I always do."

When we eat, we often follow *eating scripts*. We encounter some food situations so frequently that we develop automatic patterns or habitual behaviors to navigate them. Eating scripts are the icebergs of our diet. There are some eating scripts we are clearly aware of, but many more lurk beneath the surface of our daily activities. And whether we see them or not, they can sink our best intentions. Here are some typical scripts:

> Breakfast: Open newspaper, refill breakfast bowl and eat until finished with paper.
> Dinner: Finish eating food on plate, take additional helpings until others are done.
> Snack: Find cable movie to watch, make popcorn.

We all have breakfast scripts, snacking scripts, restaurant scripts, beverage scripts, cooking scripts, plate-cleaning scripts, and so on. We also have scripts that tell us when it's time to stop eating. In fact, if you were to ask a number of people what it was that caused them to stop eating, only some of them would say, "I was full." Others would say they stopped when they ran out of time or when their eating companions were through.[1] Still others would say they stopped when the food was gone, when their television program was over, or when they'd finished whatever they were reading. This can be dangerous to the waistline. If we eat until the food is gone or until we're through reading, the family-size box of Frosted Cheerios and the Sunday newspaper are not going to be a winning combination.

Here's where reengineering your environment comes in. We can change gain-weight scripts into lose-weight scripts. We can turn our saboteurs into our allies. Let's start with our family and friends.

Family, Friends, and Fat

One of life's great pleasures is to share food with family and friends. What we don't always realize is how strongly our family and friends influence what we eat. When we're with people we enjoy, we often lose track of how much we're eating. We eat longer than we otherwise would, and we let others set the pace for how fast and how much we eat.

Why does eating with other people make us lose track of how much we eat? In the excitement of the conversation, we forget whether we ate two bread rolls or three, or whether we had seconds or thirds of the pasta. We're so involved with our friends or family, that the whole idea of monitoring what's going into our mouths is strange. We know we ate, but we don't know how much.

When we're with people we like, we tend to eat for longer than when we're by ourselves. We're having fun, and we want to hear a funny story, or to tell one. Furthermore, it's just good manners to wait until everyone has finished before we push away from the table. At some point (clearly after high school), we develop enough empathy not to want to leave someone eating by themselves. So we nibble a bit more on the salad, or have another piece of bread. Maybe we decide to have dessert along with some of the others. Eating is like shopping: the longer you stay at the mall, the more you buy. Just so—the longer you stay at the table, the more you tend to eat.

Rescripting Your Dinner

- Try to be the last person to start eating.
- Pace yourself with the slowest eater at the table.
- Avoid the "just one more helping" request (and temptation) by always leaving some food on your plate as if you're still eating.
- Preregulate consumption by deciding how much to eat prior to the meal instead of during the meal.

Psychology professor John DeCastro has shown that this chow-down tendency is so strong, it's almost mathematically predictable. On average, if you eat with one other person, you'll eat about 35 percent more than you otherwise would. If you eat with a group of seven or more, you'll eat nearly twice as much—96 percent more—than you would if you were eating alone at the Thanksgiving card table in the other room. If you get a reservation for a table for four, you'll end up right in the middle—you'll eat about 75 percent more calories than if you reserve a table for one.[2]

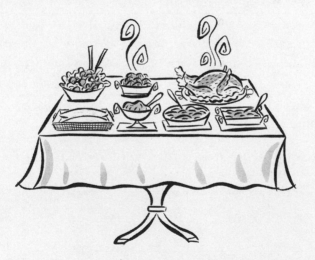

Our friends and family influence us by setting the pace for the meal. When we're with others, we tend to mimic the speed at which they eat and how much they eat. There are a number of snack experiments in which someone is invited in for an afternoon snack of cookies, and they "happen" to find themselves with a second person, who also showed up for the snack. Little do they know that the second person is actually an undercover "pacesetter" who has been secretly instructed to eat either six cookies, three cookies, or one cookie. What is always found is that the more cookies this pacesetter eats, the more cookies the unsuspecting snacker eats. The pacesetter eats one, the snacker eats one. The pacesetter eats six, the snacker eats five or six.[3]

In another clever study, researchers set up a series of lunches featuring three of the basic American food groups: pizza, cookies, and soft drinks.[4] The people who were invited were first asked to eat alone; on a subsequent occasion they were placed in groups of four or eight.

When people ate alone, some ate very little and others ate quite a lot. What was interesting was what those same people did when eating with others. When eating in groups of four or eight, light eaters ate more, and heavy eaters ate less. This goes back to the power of norms. Large groups

How Much More Your Friends Make You Eat

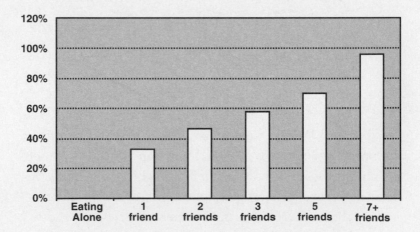

create their own norms for pizza consumption. If everyone else is eating three pieces of pizza, and you were going to eat just one, you might find yourself nibbling on a second piece. Similarly, if you would otherwise have eaten six, you might find yourself slowing down, showing a rare display of restraint and eating only five. When you eat with a group, the average amount others eat suggests the amount that's appropriate for you to eat. The pace subtly influences us.

How can you use this information? If you're trying to lose weight, go to lunch with your Atkins'-approved friends, not with the crowd that is going out for three-cheese deep-dish pizza. Also, sit next to slow eaters, who can help you pace your eating, not the speed eaters who eat like they grew up in a family of 12.

Let's say you have a one-hour lunch break. You can either choose to eat for an hour alone or in a group. If you're trying to lose weight, what should you do?

It depends. If you tend to be a heavy eater, you should eat with the group. If you're a lighter eater, you should eat by yourself.

Birds of a feather eat together. This may be one contributing reason why couples and families tend to be similar sizes. That is, some families are skinny and some families are not. If there's a majority of overweight people in a family, the frequency, quantity, and time spent eating puts more pressure on a person who's trying to lose weight. Weight can be inherited, but it can also be contagious.

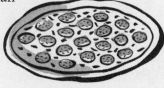

Eating Scripts of the Manly Man

Do you always eat more when you eat with other people? Not always. People who are at job-interview lunches or who are eating with an unfamiliar client or boss tend to undereat because they're self-conscious and want to make a good impression.[5] Dating, too, is a special case.

In one of our movie popcorn studies, we singled out dating couples and asked them whether they paid attention to how much popcorn they ate while watching the movie. We also weighed their buckets to see how much they had eaten.

If you pay attention to how much you eat during a movie, will you eat more or will you eat less than if you mindlessly munch away? It seems reasonable you would eat less, and in fact, this is exactly what was found with the women in our study. The more closely a woman on a date said she paid attention to how much she ate, the less she ate.

Not so with the men. In fact, it was the exact opposite. The more a male indicated that he paid attention to how much he ate, the *more* he ate. This seems to make no sense—unless you factor in the power of gender roles and expectations.

These same females indicated on these surveys that to "overeat" would not be considered feminine. With males it was quite different. For them, a healthy appetite—or, as one put it, being "insatiable"—was a sign of being manly. In our follow-up interviews, several even used words like "studly" and "powerful."

So men and women had opposite eating scripts for a date. Women thought it was more attractive and feminine to eat less. Guys thought it was studly and masculine to show they have voracious, healthy appetites, like real men should. Some of them ate more than they otherwise would have because they thought they were impressing their girlfriends with their macho eating behavior.

Imagine a hypothetical dinner-and-movie date between Brad and Barb. After our movie-theater experiment we wrote two descriptions of a date that were identical, except in one version Brad ate "a couple handfuls" of his popcorn and in the other version he ate "almost all of his popcorn." Seventy college males were given the first description to read and seventy were given the second. Even though the rest of the

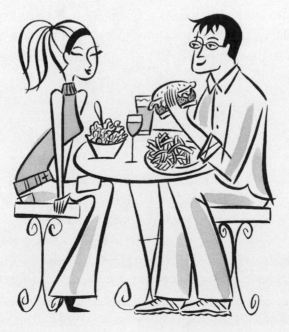

story about Brad and what he did on his date was rich with distracting detail, men who read the version where Brad ate most of his popcorn consistently rated him as stronger, more aggressive, and more masculine than those who read the version in which he ate just a few handfuls.

Then we took this a step further. We asked, "How much weight (in pounds) do you think Brad can bench-press?" If he had eaten all of the popcorn, our participants estimated he could bench-press an average of 21 more pounds.[6]

So does Brad's Macho-Man-Savage appetite impress the ladies? We did this same study with 140 college women. While the manly eating Brad may have been impressive to his male readers, his charm was lost on the ladies. They didn't think he was any stronger, more aggressive, or more masculine than the "couple handfuls" version of Brad. He also wasn't any more of a bench-pressing stud-muffin.

There are a lot of things we guys do to impress women. Eating all of our popcorn at the movies is probably one we can cross off our list.

All-You-Can-Eat Television

It's about as close to an established fact as things get in the social sciences: People who watch a lot of TV are more likely to be overweight than people who don't. The less TV people watch, the skinnier they are.[7] It doesn't matter if they're 14 or 44. It doesn't matter if they watch network TV, cable TV, the Food Network, or the NASCAR Network. As TV viewing goes up, weight goes up, and there are good reasons why. People who watch a lot of TV exercise less and they eat more. Both children and adults tend to snack more when watching television, and they do so even if they are not physically hungry.[8] In fact, people who snack while watching TV rate themselves as being less hungry than those who snack when they're *not* watching television.[9]

TV is a triple eating threat. Aside from leading you to eat, it leads you to not pay attention to how much you eat, and it leads you to eat for too long. It's a scripted, conditioned ritual—we turn on the TV, we sit down in our favorite spot, we salivate, and we go get a snack. Eating or drinking gives us something to do with our hands and it occupies us while we focus on the plot of our television show and on the questions it raises: "What else is on?" "Have I seen this one before?" "Did the Flintstones really happen?" And because our stomachs can't count, the more we focus on what we're watching, the more we end up forgetting how much we've eaten.[10]

One weekend our Lab invited students in to see the TV pilot *Hazzard County,* which was intended to be a *Dukes of Hazzard* spin-off with fewer car chases and a less complex plot. We showed them either a half hour of the show or a full hour's worth. We gave each person in both groups a large bowl of popcorn and a large dish of baby carrots. The longer they watched TV, the more they ate. In fact, if they watched TV for an hour, they ate 28 percent more popcorn than if they watched for a half hour. If there's good news here, it's that they also ate slightly more (11 percent more) carrots. So it seems that time discriminates against no food.

Okay, TV can make you fat. But our more literary friends are not safe either. Their newspapers will make them fatter if they pour an extra bowl of breakfast cereal while they read

Meal Multi-tasking

Ever eaten breakfast while you're weaving in and out of traffic? It's called "dashboard dining," and the roads are jammed with these diners. Meal multi-tasking—eating while doing something else, like driving, working, watching TV, or reading—is popular. A recent poll of 1,521 people found that:

91% typically watch TV when eating meals at home
62% are sometimes or often too busy to sit down and eat
35% eat lunch at their desk while they work
26% often eat when driving

Anything that takes our focus off the food makes us more likely to overeat without knowing it. Dashboard diners and desktop diners are less likely to be overachievers than they are to be overeaters.[11]

the editorial page. This book will make you fatter if you can't finish this chapter without reaching for a snack.

The same is true with the radio. In one study, people who listened to a lunchtime radio mystery show ate 15 percent more than those who didn't.[12] The basic rule: distractions of all kinds make us eat, forget how much we eat, and extend how long we eat—even when we're not hungry.

All of our eating scripts are reinforced by the power of habit. In one clever study, Paul Rozin showed that amnesiac patients who were told it was dinnertime ate a second complete meal within 30 minutes after having eaten a prior meal.[13] Even though they couldn't have been physically hungry, simply thinking it was time to have a meal or a snack was enough to make them eat.

The tendency to use a clock to tell yourself when you're hungry seems to be especially strong for people who are overweight. The late Stanley Schachter did a *Candid Camera*–worthy study on this topic. He and his team put obese and normal-weight individuals in windowless rooms for a full day with all the food they could eat. In the room was a clock that was designed to run faster than a normal clock. When it was 10 A.M., the clock would indicate it was noon. Whereas normal-weight individuals tended to rely on their "internal clock" and eat when they were hungry, the obese individuals tended to focus on the clock on the wall. If it said 12:00, it was time for lunch. If it said 6:00, it was time for dinner. The obese participants' meals were just as big as those given to the normal-weight participants, but in real time they were eating much more frequently.[14]

Slow Italian and Fast Chinese

Where do you want to eat tomorrow night—the Italian Patio or the Chinese Garden? Regardless of what you order, your choice of restaurant will influence how long you eat, how fast you eat, and how much you eat. The Italian Patio has soft music, subtle wood tones, and candlelight. The Chinese Garden greets you with bright fluorescent lights, random yellows and reds, and a scratchy speaker playing Shanghai Muzak a little too loud. Which one should you pick if you're on a diet?

The definitive answer is "It depends."

The atmosphere of a restaurant can cause you to overeat if it gets you to stay longer (thus ordering and eating more), or if it gets you to eat faster. It's difficult to wolf your way through a meal that's lit by candles and indirect lights. Soft lighting calms us and makes us more comfortable and disinhibited. We linger long enough to consider an unplanned dessert or an extra drink. On the other hand, when the light is bright, we tend to gulp and go. This can mean that by the time we start feeling full, we've already overeaten.

Music has a similar effect. When it's soft and pleasantly familiar, we feel happier, more relaxed, and more likely to stick around. Make that music a little too loud or a little too irritating, and you're out of there as soon as possible.

How do we know this? A few years ago, marketing professor Ronald Milliman ran an interesting study in the Dallas, Texas, area. He convinced a nice restaurant to experiment with their dinnertime background music, testing faster, upbeat tracks against soft, relaxing instrumentals. The owners were easy to convince. On weekends the restaurant was packed beyond capacity. If fast music "turned tables" more quickly without costing them profits, fast music it would be. Over eight weekends they alternated between fast and slow music, and Milliman tracked how long 1,392 of their patrons ate and how much they spent.[15]

Owners, waiters, diners, lend me your ears. With pleasant, slow, semi-familiar music playing in the restaurant, diners stuck around 11 minutes longer (56 minutes total) than did diners on the fast-music nights. While they did not spend more money on food, the average slow-music table spent over $30 on drinks, far more than the $21.62 spent by the fast-music group. What was the soft music worth? An extra 41 percent in drink revenues per table.

But before you head out for a stay-trim meal at the light, bright, noisy red-and-gold-leaf Chinese Garden, be forewarned. In this type of environment, you are likely to eat a lot faster. And because you "speed eat," you will probably eat more than you want. Remember the 20-Minute Rule: by the time your stomach sends a "full" signal, you have already filled and eaten another plate from the buffet.

None of this will be news to restaurant designers. Fast-food restaurants want you in and out of there so more people can take your place. They decorate for speed eating: bright lights, lots of hard surfaces that reflect lots of noise, and a high contrast, high arousal yellow-and-red color scheme.[16]

What about the white tablecloth dinner at The Normandy restaurant or at Joe Gantz Steak House? You can bet that the lights will be low, the music soft, the colors muted, and the waitstaff will be attentive and will be "up-selling" desserts and drinks throughout the meal. You can also bet that you will order and eat more than you planned.

Some people think we linger at upscale restaurants and eat more at them because the food is so good. They think that the quality of the food matters more than the atmosphere. It should come as no surprise that this has been tested.

For a *20/20* television episode on "Portion Distortion," my Food and Brand Lab did a Cinderella makeover on a Hardee's restaurant in Champaign, Illinois.[17] The main room had the bright lights, bright colors, and loud noise typical of fast-food restaurants. But we took what had been

Restaurant Rules: Enjoy More and Eat Less

- If the breadbasket is on the table, you're going to eat bread. Either ask the waiter to take it away early or keep it on the other side of the table.
- Portion sizes are often ample—split an entrée, have half packed to take home, or simply order two appetizers instead.
- While soft music and candlelight can improve your enjoyment of a meal, remember that they can make you eat more if you linger, and prompt you to give in to the temptation of dessert or another drink.
- If you want dessert, see if someone will share it with you. The best part of a dessert is the first two bites.
- Establish a Pick-Two rule: appetizer, drink, dessert—pick any two.

a separate smoking room and brought in plants and paintings, shades and indirect lights, and we put white tablecloths and candles on the tables. We topped it off by soundproofing the room and piping in smooth jazz. When lunchtime customers arrived at Hardee's, they ordered as they normally would. They went to the counter, looked at the menu board, and typically selected a meal-deal that came with a sandwich, fries, and a drink that they could freely refill at a fountain machine on the left side of the counter.

After each group of customers (usually two or four people) ordered, they were either seated in the main part of the restaurant or were escorted to the converted dining room. They were told it was a new idea the restaurant was trying.

If they were seated in the converted dining room, their food was delivered to them and a waiter frequently stopped by to refill their beverage and to ask them if they wanted anything else.

Even though most people were on their lunch break and needed to return to work, those in the relaxing atmosphere lingered and ate for 11 minutes longer than those in the main eating area. Although the diners in the renovated room often ordered desserts, they compensated by eating less of their sandwiches and French fries, and drinking less of their beverages. After they finished their meal, they rated the food as tasting better than did the diners in the loud, colorful, main dining room. They also said they would be more likely to come back within the month.

The candlelight and soft music at the white-tablecloth restaurant are no more an accident than the bright red-and-yellow motif at the fast-food franchise down the street. Not only do we expect those sights and sounds, but they serve an important purpose for the restaurant. So does another one of our senses.

Follow Your Nose

If you drive past 35th and Market Street in Philadelphia, it's hard to not notice the huge brass nose and lips on the south side of the street. It looks like someone went to Mount Rushmore, bronzed George Washington's nose, and then—thinking no one would notice—cut it off with a blowtorch and moved it into exile in West Philadelphia.

This is the home of the internationally renowned Monell

Chemical Senses Center. It's also home to hundreds of white rats in cages and to dozens of white-coated scientists in labs. One of the Center's many areas of expertise is the investigation of how smells and tastes influence our food preferences.[18] For example, Monell researchers Julie Mennella and Gary Beauchamp showed that simply having pregnant women drink carrot juice in their last trimester significantly increased how much their babies preferred carrot-flavored cereal months later.[19]

Marketers already know that odors are linked with taste and craving. Consider what the researchers in my Lab call "the Cinnabon Effect." Successful marketing is about positive associations and memory, and smell is hardwired to memory. Cinnabon has this nailed. Cinnabon stores are positioned beside stores that don't sell food, so there's no smell competition. As a result, you can walk through the mall feeling perfectly fine, but once you catch that first whiff of Cinnabon goodness wafting through the air, you're hooked.

You either have to hold your breath like an underwater swimmer and keep moving until you run out of air, or you have to stop by for a taste. That smell was worth approximately $200 million in sales in 2003.[20]

The French are fond of saying, "You taste first with your eyes," but it's your nose that gets your stomach revved up. If your last cold didn't convince you, try eating something you really like (say freshly baked cookies) and pinching your nose shut. They don't taste quite so great. Of course, this also works in the reverse. When children have to eat something they don't like (squash, liver, or Alka-Seltzer), they hold their nose so they can gulp it down.

Smell is big business. There are companies that exist solely because they can infuse (the word they oddly use is "impregnate") odors into plastics. This is because odor can't reliably be infused into food. Sometimes it doesn't last; at other times it changes the shelf stability of the food itself. But if you infuse the odor into packaging, it's a different story. Some day you might heat up your frozen microwavable apple pie and smell the rich apple pie aroma. Even if it's the container that you're smelling, you're primed to enjoy that apple pie even before you put your fork in. But will the smell cause you to eat more?

To examine this, we treated 24 people to a free breakfast each Wednesday morning for three weeks. Everyone ate oatmeal out of three different bowls on three different weeks in three different orders. On week one, some were given plain oatmeal in a normal bowl. The next week, the oatmeal was in a bowl made of plastic that had been manufactured to smell like cinnamon-and-raisin. The final week, they were given a bowl impregnated with the smell of macaroni and cheese. We wanted to find out whether adding the artificial odors would change how much people ate.

This study was one I was conducting with Armand Cardello at the U.S. Army Research Labs at Natick, Massachusetts. The objective was to see whether we could stimulate troops in the field to increase food consumption when deployed in a combat situation.[21] When deployed, troops can burn anywhere from 3,000 to 6,000 calories a day. They need to eat—a lot. But in these situations, all sorts of smells—those of diesel fuel and so on—can make food taste less than appetizing. Our work with smell enhancers was aimed at seeing how we could overcome these competing odors.

The first step was to see if they worked at all in a more low-key setting. That is, a lab where people didn't have to smell diesel fuel and wear helmets while they ate breakfast.

What we found was that smell made a big difference. Adding a nice cinnamon-and-raisin smell to our plain-tasting oatmeal led people to eat more. Adding an inconsistent odor—macaroni and cheese—got them to eat notably less. Even though it didn't change the taste of the food, the sensory confusion put a real damper on their appetite.

When working with the Army as a scientist, everything is on a need-to-know basis. I needed to know the problem, and I needed to help find a solution. With my level of security clearance, however, I did *not* need to know what the Army would do with the results, so this is where the story ends. But whether or not scented bowls find their way into the Army, I bet they find their way into the microwave section of our grocery stores before too long. Mmm . . . smells like homemade apple pie.

The power of the smell–appetite connection has not been lost on the supermodel world. If a smell can help make you feel full or sated or satisfied, it also can be used to curb cravings until they pass. It's not uncommon for supermodels to buy a candy bar, take a bite, chew it, and spit it out.[22] Some even keep the wrapper, so they can smell it for a fix.

Check the Weather Forecast

California is the Golden State. It's the land of beautiful beaches and beautiful people. People like me from the blizzard states of the Midwest love to attribute the hard, trim California beach bodies to the fact that California weather allows people to be outside moving and exercising constantly. After all, most people lose a little bit of weight in the summer and gain it in the winter because we're more active in the summer and we're burning more calories.

A deeper explanation is related to the air temperature and to our need to keep our core body temperature constant.

Our benevolent metabolism wants to help us stay alive, and it does so by using food and liquid to either warm us up or cool us down. In the middle of a cold January night, we need more energy to warm and maintain our core body temperature, so our body tells us to eat more, and it even speeds up our digestion so we'll feel hungry sooner.[23] In the middle of a hot August afternoon, the body needs more liquids to cool and maintain its core temperature, so it tells us to drink more. As a result, we might lose weight in the summer because we're moving around more, but we also lose weight because we're eating less and drinking more water.[24]

Now, what about spring and fall? In general—not counting springtime swimsuit diets—most Northern Hemisphere people eat more in the fall than in the spring. It might be because the falling temperature signals our bodies to fatten up for winter, but another provocative explanation has been suggested.

In 2004, I presented some of my research findings to a group of biologists and psychologists at the Max Planck Institutes in Germany. While world-renowned for their Nobel Prize–winning work in the hard sciences, the Institutes are now becoming an international force in the social sciences.

When asked what time of year I conducted one of my studies, I was puzzled. My questioner went on to propose that our tendency to eat more in the fall than the spring may have evolutionary roots. The idea is called "evolutionary psychology," and it assumes that brains and behavior adapt across generations to ensure our survival.

A few thousand Aprils ago, food was not plentiful. Fruit was not ripe, crops were not mature, winter stores were exhausted, and the animals we hunted were either scarce, small, or emaciated from the winter. Many people starved, and the advantage went to those who could survive on less food.

In the fall, however, the fruit was mature, the harvest was in, and the deer and the antelope were chubby and had "dinner" written all over them. In almost every culture in the Northern Hemisphere, fall is the time for all-you-can-eat holidays that celebrate the harvest (Thanksgiving in the United States and Canada, Moon Festival in China, Beaujolais Day in France). It's nature's own groaning-board buffet season. Evolutionary psychology claims that our brains and appetites adapt to eating rhythms generation after generation. This contributes to why we may find ourselves eating more in the fall compared to the spring.

If the seasons cause us to eat in cycles, so—on a day-to-day basis—does the weather. We are less hungry on a hot day and more hungry on a chilly, rainy one. On those chilly, rainy days we want to eat. And the impact of weather on our growl-ing stomachs has not been lost on enterprising companies.

Consider this: Most people at home indicate that they don't decide what they're going to eat for lunch until shortly before noon. That is, at about 11:00 A.M. they start looking around or thinking about what they want to make for them-selves or their family. So, if a good suggestion on the radio were to catch their ear, it could influence what they eat. And it does.

Rainy, chilly days are made to order for a soup-and-sandwich lunch. The Campbell Soup Company knows this and they also know that the typical American household once had 11.3 cans of Campbell's soup stacked in the back of their cupboard. At one point in the 1980s, Campbell's de-veloped a series of commercials for radio stations called "storm spots."[25] These radio ads referred to the rain and pointed out that soup is a cozy, warm, comfort food; that it goes so well with sandwiches that are easy to make; and that—not coincidently—the listener probably happens to have a number of cans of Campbell's soup in the cupboard right at this minute.

Radio stations were instructed that if it were raining or storming between the hours of 10:00 A.M. and 1:00 P.M., they should play these radio ads. The expectation was that people would dutifully eat their soup and buy more the next time they went to the store.

Reengineering Strategy #5:
Create Distraction-Free Eating Scripts

As long as we believe it is food that causes us to overeat, we are lost. Television, friends, and weather seem pretty unrelated to what we eat. That's why they have such a powerful effect on us.

- **Rescript your diet danger zones.** We all have various eating scripts for the five most common diet danger zones—dinners, snacks, parties, restaurants, desks/dashboards. (See Appendix B.) A common dinner script—particularly for men—involves eating second helpings of most foods until everyone at the table is finished or until the food is gone. If such a man wanted to rescript his dinner, he might try being the last one to start eating, pacing himself with his spouse, serving triple helpings of the healthy foods and single helpings of the meat and potatoes, or not including bread. Similarly, after-work snacking could be rescripted with a stick of gum rather than whatever is in the refrigerator.
- **Distract yourself before you snack.** Distractions are good news and bad news. They are good when they prevent us from starting to snack. They are bad when they prevent us from stopping. At home, you can make your snacking life less distracting and less alluring by eating in one room only, such as the dining room or kitchen.

- **Serve yourself before you start.** If you can't distract yourself from a yummy snack, you can minimize the damage it does in a distracting situation (such as eating in front of the TV). To avoid "eating until it's over," dish yourself out a ration before you start. Eating straight from a box, bag, or serving bowl is the recipe for regret.

6

The Name Game

WE KNOW WHAT WE like, right?

Not as much as we think we do. Our "taste" resides in our head as well as in our mouth. We often taste what we *think* we will taste. In the same way that mindless eating can lead us to overeat, our expectations about the taste of a food can "trick our taste buds," making us think a food tastes much better or worse than it actually does.[1]

Knowing how this works is a big deal if you are a $200,000-a-year chef, a Navy cook, a brand manager, or a food critic. It's also a big deal if you're a mother who is trying to encourage her family to eat their vegetables, a Food Network fan, or a weekend party cook who wants people to love the food you make.

Eating in the Dark

Although the guards who stop you at the sentry post are well armed—at one time with 30-caliber machine guns—

this isn't the Pentagon or a secret mountain bunker. It's the U.S. Army Natick Soldier Center, tucked away in the quiet town of Natick, Massachusetts, about 15 miles west of Boston. In these labs, the U.S. Army does most of the research on what soldiers eat, what they should eat, and how to get them to eat more of it. When it comes to soldier welfare and effectiveness, food gets elevated to an issue of national security.

In addition to the sensory experts who run the Natick Labs, a *Who's Who* list of researchers from Finland, England, France, and the United States has pilgrimaged there to brainstorm and conduct studies. Many will examine how colors, wrappers, expiration dates, labeled ingredients, logos, and packaging change what soldiers think of the taste of food and how much they eat.[2]

Here's the problem: When soldiers are first deployed in a combat situation, they're often overworked and overstressed, but they tend to undereat. Even when they are given plenty of food and plenty of time to eat it, they simply don't eat enough and they begin losing weight. Some of those studies with colors, wrappers, and packaging are aimed at tricking a soldier's taste buds into liking a food and eating enough of it to stay alert and strong.

Take the case of eating in the dark. Soldiers in the field frequently have to eat without lights, and they don't always know exactly what they're eating. How does this affect their sense of taste?

When I was on sabbatical there in 2004, this was one of the questions we tackled. Alan Wright and I invited 32 Natick Lab employees (in squad-size groups of eight) to rate the taste of some new strawberry yogurts the Army was testing. We told them we wanted to make sure the food tasted good even if it couldn't be seen.

Then we turned out the lights in the lab.

And we did not give them strawberry yogurt. We gave them chocolate yogurt. It didn't seem to matter very much. The mere suggestion that they were eating strawberry yogurt led 19 of 32 people to rate it as having a good strawberry taste. One even said that strawberry yogurt was her favorite yogurt and this would be her new favorite brand.[3] Soldiers, just like us, use all sorts of cues or signals to help taste food. One of these is our eyesight. If it doesn't look like strawberry, it doesn't taste like strawberry. But another important cue is the name of a food. If we can't see the food and someone tells us we're going to taste strawberry, we taste strawberry, even if it's really chocolate.

A rose may be a rose by any other name. But this isn't true with food. Except in extreme cases, we taste what we think we will taste.

They Call the Jell-O Yellow

That's right. Lemon Jell-O is yellow. Billy disagrees.

Billy had one of the toughest cooking jobs in the world. He could only order food and cooking supplies once every four months. He and his adopted family couldn't leave and eat anywhere else for those entire four months. Nearly every member of his family was overworked, overstressed, and fearing for their lives. There were also around 900 of them, almost all males between 18 and 30.

Billy was a World War II Navy cook, and we corresponded when our Lab was conducting a large-scale survey of how the war had changed the food habits of those involved in it.[4] He was a true Iron Chef. From Pearl Harbor to Midway, Billy was in charge of keeping a shipload of sailors happy for three meals a day. He learned tricks to make that happen.

On what turned out to be one particularly long tour, Billy discovered that he had accidentally ordered twice as much lemon Jell-O as he needed, but no cherry Jell-O. Small things can make a big difference when people are under stress, and sure enough, two months out, some sailors began complaining that there was no cherry Jell-O. On one occasion, a fight broke out over this. There were pointed remarks that such carelessness should result in Billy being reprimanded or even demoted.

In the face of growing rebellion, Billy got creative. He made lemon Jell-O as usual, but added red food coloring to it. Of course it was still lemon-flavored, but it looked like cherry Jell-O.

When it was served, no one thought differently. Some sailors even complimented him on finally finding the cherry Jell-O. He served the red lemon Jell-O twice more before returning to port and restocking. No one suspected what happened. By simply coloring the Jell-O, Billy gave sailors the opportunity to taste what they expected to taste.

Why can we be so easily and mindlessly fooled when it comes to taste? Psychologists call this "expectation assimilation" and "confirmation bias." In the case of food, it means that our taste buds are biased by our imagination. Basically, if you expect a food to taste good, it will. At the very least, it will taste better than if you had thought it would only be so-so.

But expectation assimilation also works in the opposite direction. If you expect a food to taste bad, it will.

Billy probably couldn't explain the psychology behind his Jell-O trick, but he intuitively knew it would work. "Seeing red" was enough to transform lemon to cherry.

Changing Jell-O colors may seem like a trivial point, but it is not. Exactly the same principle is at work in every fine restaurant and with every home kitchen gourmet. That principle is called "presentation."

While the French say "We taste first with our eyes," the Japanese talk about *katachi no aji,* which means "the shape of the taste." Expensive-looking gold-trimmed plates, exotic shavings of garnish, artsy squiggles of sauce from squirt bottles . . . all of these pique our expectations that the food will taste great. And they work.

Consider the power of plates alone. At the end of lunchtime in the Bevier Cafeteria, in Urbana, Illinois, 175 people were given a free brownie dusted with powdered sugar. They were told it was a new recipe that the cafeteria was thinking of adding to the dessert section, and they were asked what they thought of it and how much they would be willing to pay for it. Every brownie was the same size and from the same recipe. The one difference was the way it was presented. Some were handed their brownie on a snow white piece of china; others were given their brownie on a paper plate; and the rest were given it on a paper napkin.

Those who were presented their brownie on china claimed this new brownie recipe was excellent. A number of them even commented on the efforts the chef was making to up-grade the cafeteria. Those who had eaten their brownie off the paper plate said the brownie was "good." Those who were served their brownie on the napkin rated it as "okay, but nothing special."

How much is this information worth to a cafeteria that sells 12,000 brownies a year? To find out, we asked these same people how much they would pay for the brownie they ate. The people who were served the brownie on china said they would be willing to pay an average of $1.27. Paper-plate brownies averaged 76¢, while those eating off a napkin said they would pay only 53¢ for the same taste experience.[5] The difference between the china brownie and the napkin brownie is 74¢, which translates to almost $9,000 a year. That buys a lot of nice dishes.

Menu Magic

Smart restaurant owners know that the difference between profit and loss can take place before the food is even ordered.[6] This is why they craft and recraft the décor, lighting, music, and table settings to create positive expectations. They also harness the power of the pen by using descriptive, tasty words.

We see this in all kinds of successful restaurants—low end to high end. Take menu names. For under $5, you can buy a Black Angus Monster Burger, Cheese Lover's Delight Personal Pan Pizza, a Baja Fiesta Taco value meal, and the genuine genius of them all, a McDonald's Happy Meal.

In the middle of the eating spectrum, restaurant chains give their foods names such as Jack Daniels® Chicken, Psychedelic Sorbet®, or the Bloomin' Onion®. On the white tablecloth end of the culinary spectrum, Tennyson and Keats wannabes come up with names like Boeuf Provençal en Gelée.

A few years back, a menu in a French-style restaurant in the Hanover, New Hampshire, area described one dish as being "graced with spring-fresh medallions of well-mannered beef." Well-mannered beef? Are there cows out there who say, "I realize I'm six hours away from becoming an entrée, but I'm okay with that. Enough about me. How are you doing?" Doubtful. Yet if these menu names and descriptions seem so ridiculous out of context, why are they so common?

They are common because they *work*. They work in two ways. First, they entice us to buy the food. Second, they lead us to expect it will taste good, which pretty much pre-programs our taste buds.

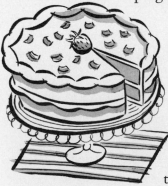

Consider two pieces of day-old chocolate cake. If one is named "chocolate cake," and the other is named "Belgian Black Forest Double Chocolate Cake," people will buy the second. That's no surprise. What's more interesting is that after trying it, people will rate it as tasting better than an identical piece of "plain old cake." It doesn't even matter that the Black Forest is not in Belgium.

We know this is true because we tested it in the real world.

Which Menu Has the Better Food?

MENU A	MENU B
• Red Beans with Rice	• Traditional Cajun Red Beans with Rice
• Seafood Filet	• Succulent Italian Seafood Filet
• Grilled Chicken	• Tender Grilled Chicken
• Chicken Parmesan	• Home-Style Chicken Parmesan
• Chocolate Pudding	• Satin Chocolate Pudding
• Zucchini Cookies	• Grandma's Zucchini Cookies

Back to the Bevier Cafeteria. Cafeteria food, like school hot lunches, has its share of image problems. This particular cafeteria was trying to enhance its image while also encouraging people to buy more of their vegetable side dishes and healthier foods. How could this be done? By changing the names of the foods.

We took six different foods—vegetables, main dishes, and

low-fat desserts—and offered them on different days. Sometimes they had their boring, basic name and sometimes they had a slightly more descriptive name. Every day for six weeks we rotated these foods on and off the menu so no one would become suspicious. One day Red Beans and Rice would be offered, and two weeks later it would reappear as *Traditional Cajun* Red Beans with Rice. One week you could buy the *Succulent Italian* Seafood Filet for $2.90; the next week the Seafood Filet was available at the same price. Exact same food; slightly different names.[7]

Anybody who bought one of the six foods—either labeled or unlabeled—was discreetly observed while they ate. When they were close to being finished, they were given a half-page survey that asked them to rate the food and the cafeteria. There were a number of interesting discoveries.

First, the foods with descriptive names sold 27 percent more.[8] And even though they were priced exactly the same, the customers who ate them consistently rated them as a better value than did the people who ate the same dishes with the boring old names.

But what about the taste? A nice name might lead to raving expectations, but can't it also lead to a backlash? "Succulent Italian Seafood Filet . . . no way, this tastes more like a dry fishstick!" After all, truth be told, the food was nothing special.

Not so. The foods with descriptive names were rated as more appealing and tastier than the identical foods with the less attractive labels. Furthermore, when asked what they thought about the foods, the diners eating the descriptive foods tended to claim that they were "fantastic" or "great recipes."

What's on Today's Hot Lunch Menu?

A peek at the hot lunch menus from two schools gives us an idea of what awaits the next generation of Italian food lovers.[9]

PHILLIPS EXETER ACADEMY	PHILIP HIGH SCHOOL
Exeter, New Hampshire	Philip, South Dakota
1,050 students	885 people—in the town
$34,500 tuition for	$31,103 average household
boarding school (2006)	income (2000)
"Huc venite, pueri,	"Home of the mighty
ut viri sitis"	Philip Scotties"
MENU (2-13-06)	MENU (2-13-06)
White bean soup	Pizza
Homemade tomato olive bread	Corn
Baked ziti	Peach
Honey dipped fried chicken	Milk
Spinach tomato rice	
Caesar salad	

Yet something else was found that was of particular interest to the cafeteria. The customers who ate the food with descriptive names had more favorable attitudes toward the cafeteria as a whole. Some commented that it was trendy and up-to-date. Others thought the chef was probably classically trained, perhaps in Europe. Again, the foods were exactly alike. The only difference was the addition of one or two descriptive words. These one or two words changed sales, tastes, and attitudes toward the restaurant.

Nowhere is menu magic more common than at the

top-end restaurants. Why? Perhaps because people who own, manage, and cook in these restaurants are very serious about their food, and they have vocabularies to match. They use vivid adjectives to trigger our expectations, often drawing on one or more of four basic themes:

1. **Geographic Labels:** Words that create an image or ideology of a geographic area associated with the food. Think Southwestern Tex-Mex Salad, Iowa Pork Chops, Kansas City Barbeque, or Country Peach Tart.
2. **Nostalgic Labels:** Alluding to the past can trigger happy associations of family, tradition, national origin, and wholesomeness. Remember Classic Old-World Manicotti, Legendary Chocolate Mousse Pie, Green Gables Matzo Ball Soup, and Grandma's Chicken Fricassee?
3. **Sensory Labels:** Describing the taste, smell, and mouth feel of the menu item can raise expectations. Dessert chefs accomplish this masterfully—note names like Velvety Chocolate Mousse—but main-course items also benefit, such as Hearty Sizzling Steaks, Snappy Seasonal Carrots, and Buttery Plump Pasta.
4. **Brand Labels:** The idea of cross-promotions is not new, but it's now catching on fast in the chain and franchise restaurant world. They essentially tell us, "If you love the brand, you'll love this menu item." That's why we can buy Black Angus® Beef Burgers, Jack Daniels® Glazed Ribs, and Butterfinger® Blizzards. At high-end restaurants, this translates into Kobe Beef Kabob or the Niman Ranch Pork Loin.

Does such labeling ever backfire? Does anyone eat the Belgian Black Forest Double Chocolate Cake and say: "Ugh, this is just that dried old stuff left over from yesterday"? Oddly enough, it doesn't seem to happen except in almost laughably extreme instances. If the food is reasonably good, it will nearly always benefit from these descriptions.

Of course, most restaurants that stay in business do so because they are not in the habit of disappointing people. Renaming yesterday's goulash Royal Hungarian Top Sirloin Blend may generate a first-time sale, but it may also be the last. A restaurant that makes a habit of tricking customers into buying something they don't like probably won't be listed in next year's Yellow Pages.

Brand-Name Psychosis

There is actually a soft drink bottled and sold in central Pennsylvania called "*It* Cola." *It* tastes like Coca-Cola but costs less than half as much. If you go to a convenience store in Gettysburg, you can pay either $1.20 for a 20-ounce bottle of Coke or 45¢ for a 20-ounce bottle of *It*. I saved 75¢ and in a "close your eyes and try this" taste test, *It* tasted about the same as Coke to the colleague I was with.

Is Coke worried about losing market share in the Gettysburg metropolitan area? No. There are lots of people still willing to shell out the extra 75¢ to drink the "Real Thing" instead of the "*It* Thing." When they see a Coke label, they expect the soft drink to taste good. They take a sip and it does taste good. When they see an *It* label, they expect the cola to taste not-so-good, and as a result, it does.

Brand names like Coke, Snickers, Frosted Flakes, Frito-Lay, and Ben & Jerry's all have a big advantage over store

The Other Iron Chef

In the December 2004 issue of *New Scientist* magazine, Graham Lawton wrote a humorous interview article on some of our findings, titled "Angelic Host."[10] In it, he reported how cues—like names, plating, candles, and soft music—can be used to make dinner guests think they are having a great holiday meal.

Toward the end of the interview with me, he confessed to a unique cue of his own. While his guests enjoy wine and appetizers in the living room, he excuses himself to "prepare the rest of the meal." Now, the meal has pretty much been prepared for three hours, but if his guests didn't believe he was slaving away on it, they wouldn't think it was going to be very good. He simply retires to the kitchen for 15 minutes with his wine and occasionally bangs his iron pots around.

He sounds busy → he must be working hard → this will be a great meal → it is!

brands like Sam's Choice or President's Club. Once the labels are off, however, it's probably a toss-up which brand is best. A number of studies have tested popular brand names next to inexpensive store brands. Some even enlist people who claim to be 100 percent loyal to a brand, such as Frito-Lay, and then give them a number of different chips to taste and rate. Despite what they say, most people can't pick their brand once it's out of the package and into a bowl.

So why doesn't everyone buy the less expensive store brands and generic goodies? One reason is that we like to remind ourselves—and others—that we are not hopelessly cheap. We may not be able to afford a BMW, but at least we're not so destitute that we have to drink *It* Cola.

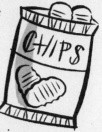

But here is the bigger reason: Most people think products with famous brand names are better. Because we think they're better, we experience them as better. It's not just the brand name, it's the advertising, the packaging, the pricing. All contribute to our positive expectations. And it works.

Nowhere is this more evident than in the so-called "sin industries" of beer, liquor, and wine. Take beer. In the age before micro-brews, differences between standard American beers were subtle, if not invisible. In a classic study, college students who claimed to be "brand loyal" beer drinkers were asked to taste and rate a number of unlabeled beers. Once the labels were removed from the beers, or once the beer was poured into a glass, all bets were off.[11] Few weekend partiers could pick their beer out of the anonymous crowd.

To date, the researchers at *Consumer Reports* have yet to engage in taste tests with different brands of vodkas. They don't need to. Since almost all unflavored vodkas are comprised only of ethyl alcohol, there probably wouldn't be any difference. The smoothness might differ, but not the taste. Still, while a generic brand charges $4 for a brain-numbing bottle, high-end brands charge over $30. How can they do so? In addition to a couple more rounds of distillation, they create a mystique with cool advertisements of icy Russian winters or with hip, high-profile bottle shapes, labels, and boxes. Indeed, the elaborate packaging for new vodkas may not just get people to order a premium brand, but dollars to rubles, it will make them think it tastes better than it actually does.

Brands also help pique our taste expectations by the way they're priced. A number of years ago, a college junior had finally been able to get a date with the woman he already dreamed he would marry. He planned to start with a picnic near a pond and then take her bowling (back when bowling was apparently romantic). He wanted to pack wine with the picnic, but on a thin budget he wasn't able to afford a bottle of Château Mouton Rothschild 1945. Instead, he selected a $1.99 screw-top bottle of Night Train Express with a black and white, semi-crooked label. Rather than being aged for decades in the cellar of a French château, it had aged on the truck on the way to the store. Knowing that a $2 bottle of wine was unlikely to impress his date, he explained his dilemma to the weekend wine clerk, who agreed to provide a new fake price label that read "$9.99."

During the picnic he elegantly unscrewed the top from the wine as he imagined James Bond or Cary Grant might have done. He then poured it into Styrofoam cups and proposed a toast. After taking a sip and wincing, the woman of his dreams picked up the bottle. Her expression changed when she saw the $9.99 label that he had so carefully left on. She said, "This is expensive. It's good."

Grape Expectations: Choosing the Right Wine

How can you select the perfect bottle of wine for a dinner party? Rest easy in the knowledge that most people can't distinguish great wine from good wine, or even pretty good wine from mediocre wine.

Most people use a two-step approach to buying wine: they choose a price level, say $10, and they then look for a bottle with a nice-looking label. Based on what we know about expectations, this makes perfect sense. If the name, origin, graphics, or shape of a wine bottle lead us to expect it will taste good, it probably *will* taste good to us.

So other than thinking twice about the North Dakota wine, try to stay away from wines named Nasti Spumante, Château West Des Moines, or Chef Boyardeaux.

Although both my date and I moved on to different vintages after graduation, we are still good friends and we still enjoy working a Night Train Express joke into an occasional conversation with each other.

Do Sweetbreads Taste Like Coffee Cake?

Great names make for great business. There are not a lot of new fish swimming in the sea or new vegetables being grown. But over the years many foods have "reinvented" themselves (think "heirloom vegetables") to fit the chic desires of the time. Just look at the menu at the next wedding dinner you attend. If you had a choice, would you choose menu A or menu B?

Menu A	Menu B
Fish Eggs	Caviar
Chinese Gooseberry	Kiwi Fruit
Snails	Escargots
Bramble	Blackberries
Calf Thymus	Sweetbreads
Chinese Moon Fruit	Pamella
Duck Liver	Foie Gras
Muttonfish	Snapper
Squid	Calamari

Even though A and B are the same foods, most of us would choose menu B, or simply drop off our wedding gift and skip the dinner. In a restaurant, we'd also be willing to pay a lot more to eat off menu B.

What a difference a name makes. Something similar happened in the 1940s. At the time, the biggest threat to American nutrition was a war—and the name of a food.

During World War II, much of America's domestic meat was being shipped overseas to feed soldiers and allies. As a result, there was a growing concern that a lengthy war would leave the United States protein-starved. The potential solution to this problem lay in what were then called organ meats: hearts, kidneys, liver, brains, stomachs, intestines, and even the feet, ears, and heads of cows, hogs, and sheep. The challenge was how to encourage Depression-era

Americans to incorporate these into their diet. To do this, the Department of Defense recruited Margaret Mead and dozens of the brightest, and subsequently most famous, psychologists, sociologists, anthropologists, food scientists, dieticians, and home economists in the nation. Their task: to make families rush to the dinner table for liverloaf and kidney pie.[12]

One of their first discoveries was that the term "organ meats" would never cause any stampedes at the meat counter. It didn't stimulate appetites, but it did stimulate imagination—in the wrong direction. Even labeling the meat case with signs saying "Succulent Italian Brain Filet" or "Traditional Cajun Tongue and Beans" was not going to be the solution.

The first step of the nutrition brain trust was to come up with the name "variety meats." Besides being less visual and more vague, it also connoted that these were meats that could be rotated into one's menu for variety and not for eternity. The names were changed in butcher shops, in cookbooks, and in government promotions. Sales increased and tastes slowly adjusted until the post-war boom in prosperity brought the choice cuts back on the table.

History repeats itself. Yesterday it was organ meats, today it is soy.

People in the soy foods industry appear mystified why many people won't eat soy foods unless forced to for health reasons. Granted, a good deal has been done to improve the taste of soy, but a lot of residual negative feelings still exist. Given the power of expectations, this is a real problem.

The National Soybean Research Center came to the Food and Brand Lab to determine why people avoid soy.[13] A series of in-depth interviews with people over the age of 40 revealed they generally had bad perceptions about the taste, aftertaste, and texture of soy foods. Some of these were due to earlier experiences with the off-taste soy filler that was used in the school hot lunch program in the 1960s and 1970s.

Still other perceptions were based on non-soy-related events. A number of people mentioned that whenever they heard the word "soy," they thought of a 1973 Charlton Heston movie—the guilty-pleasure classic *Soylent Green*. In this futuristic world, the only food source is a mysterious green substance called "soylent green." In the closing moments of the movie, Charlton Heston discovers that the source of soylent green is reconstituted humans. He stretches his arms skyward, falls to his knees, and bellows, "Soylent green is peeeoople."[14]

Despite recent improvements in the taste and texture, expectation assimilation would lead us to predict that if people expect a food with soy to taste bad, it will taste bad. But what if that food has no soy in it to begin with? If people simply believe that an ingredient is in a food, will that mindlessly influence their taste?

Our Phantom Ingredient studies were conducted in Illinois, the largest grower of soybeans in the United States. For these studies, the wrappers of 155 PowerBars were modified to say either "Contains 10 grams of protein" or "Contains 10 grams of soy protein." The only difference between the two labels was one prominent, three-letter word, "soy." In reality, there was no soy protein in this PowerBar. Exactly zero. It was a phantom ingredient. If after eating one of these PowerBars, people believed they tasted soy, they would be mindlessly responding to the power of suggestion.

People were given the bars (which were introduced as a new product) and asked to take a look at the package, and then to try them. The people who ate the bars with the label "Contains 10 grams of protein" described the bars favorably: They said they were chocolaty, chewy, and tasty. The other people, the ones who had been given the bars with "10 grams of soy protein" were not so positive.[15] Many spit out the bar, or excused themselves to get a drink of water. One man passed a piece of gum to his wife so that both could get the taste out of their mouths. When asked what they thought, they claimed that the bars had a bad aftertaste, were chalky, and didn't even taste like chocolate.

This was not good news to our soy friends. Attitudes are improving, though, and there is good precedent to think it will just take more time and more innovation.

Thirty years ago, almost none of us would've eaten something called an "unflavored bioactive dairy-based culture." But if we stirred in some fruit, sugar, flavoring, innovation, and marketing, our tastes would change. In fact, a silky lemon yogurt sounds pretty good right now.

Reengineering Strategy #6:
Create Expectations That Make You a Better Cook

Regardless whether the lemon Jell-O is cherry-colored, the fish of the day is named "Succulent Italian Seafood Filet," or the Night Train Express has a $9.99 price tag, we taste what we expect we'll taste. This is good news for those of us who barely know the recipe for toast.

- **Tell them what's for dinner.** Suppose you're asked, "What's for dinner?" *Any* two words you say will make you a better cook as long as they are positive and descriptive. Simply adding words like "traditional," "Cajun," "succulent," and "homemade" caused people in our cafeteria study to think the food tasted better and that the cook was European-trained. Big dinner party planned? The two-word technique will probably be the biggest five-minute fix to your cooking ability that you can make. What words should you use? Download a couple of restaurant menus while your oven is preheating.

- **Fix the atmosphere when you fix the food.** Spending your last 15 minutes of prep on atmospheric details will probably give you more bang than if you spend them on the food. Think soft—soft lights, soft music, soft colors. Think nice—nice plates, nice tablecloth, nice glasses. Even pizza tastes better by candlelight. Just remember to take it out of the box before you put it in the oven.

7

In the Mood for Comfort Food

NEXT TIME YOU'RE THE fifth person back in the "full shopping cart" grocery lane, glance through any three magazines in the impulse-buy rack. At least one will have an article about comfort foods or a big picture of a chocolate cake on the cover. Usually, too, it will be reinforcing one of the common comfort-food myths:

Myth #1—Most comfort foods are indulgently unhealthy.

Myth #2—People tend to eat comfort foods when they're sad, stressed, or bored.

Myth #3—Comfort food preferences become fixed when we are children.

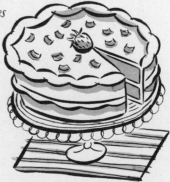

Twenty years of my research can be summarized in saying, "People's tastes are not formed by accident." But are comfort foods really this predictable? In the course of tracking down the secrets of mindless eating, our Lab has developed new insights into why we associate certain foods with comfort and when and why we eat them. First, let's start with some comfort-food myth busting.

Comfort Foods and Comfort Moods

The photos that drip off grocery store magazines would lead us to believe that the icon of comfort foods is a gooey chocolate cake stacked with ice cream and drizzled with caramel. In reality, few comfort foods are that dietetically grim. If you asked 1,004 Americans to tell you their favorite comfort food, you might be surprised. Our Lab researchers were.[1]

Although potato chips topped the list, 40 percent of the favorite comfort foods people mentioned were actually fairly healthy. They were pasta, meats, soups, main dishes, casseroles, and so on. These people not only wanted a great-for-the-moment taste of fat, salt, or sugar, they also wanted to tap in to the psychological comfort that these foods provided and the memories linked to them. Comfort foods are not always indulgent. They are the foods that feed not only our body, but also our soul.

Another surprise: When we gave people a long list of foods and asked them to rate the ones they personally found comforting, men and women might as well have been from Mars and Venus. The three foods most highly rated by females

The Most Popular Comfort Foods

	FAVORITE COMFORT FOODS	PERCENT MENTIONING ITEM AS THEIR VERY FAVORITE COMFORT FOOD
"Junk" Foods	Potato Chips	23%
	Ice Cream	14%
	Cookies	12%
	Candy / Chocolate	11%
Healthier Foods	Pasta or Pizza	11%
	Steak or Beef Burgers	9%
	Casseroles or Side Dishes	9%
	Vegetables or Salads	7%
	Soup	4%

were ice cream, chocolate, and cookies. All are sweets, and all are snack foods.

The three foods most highly rated by males were ice cream, soup, and pizza or pasta. Aside from ice cream, men rated hot foods and meal-like foods much higher than women did. The way to a man's heart appears to be more through the kitchen than through a prepackaged snack.

Why the big difference between men and women? When asked why they preferred pizza, pasta, and soup over cakes and cookies, men generally talked about how good they tasted and how filling they were. But when we probed a bit deeper, many also said that when they ate these foods they felt "spoiled," "pampered," "taken care of," or "waited on." Generally they associated these foods with being the focus of attention from either their mother or wife.

And women? Although they liked hot-meal comfort foods just fine, these foods did not carry the associations of being "spoiled," "taken care of," or "waited on." In fact, quite the opposite. When women thought of these foods, they were reminded of the work they or their mothers had to do to produce them. These foods didn't represent comfort, they represented preparation and cleanup.

For women, snacklike foods—candy, cookies, ice cream, chocolate—were hassle-free. Part of their comfort was to not have to make or clean up anything. It was both effortless and mindless eating.

What about the myth of negative moods? If we judged by daytime talk shows and diet books, we would think that most comfort foods are unhealthy foods eaten by people when they're depressed, bored, or lonely. But among the 1,004 North Americans we surveyed, we saw quite the opposite. They were more likely to seek out comfort foods

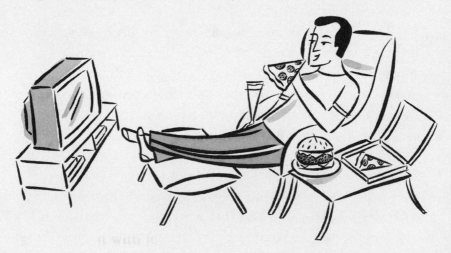

When Comfort Foods Don't Comfort

We invited 34 students in for a study break dinner during stressful mid-terms. We knew from a survey earlier in the semester that meatloaf was one of their favorite comfort foods. Seventeen of them were going to be served a nice meatloaf dinner. We wanted to see if it would reduce their stress level more than the others who would be served a burrito dinner, which they also liked but which they didn't consider a comfort food.

The meatloaf worked its magic—but not for everyone. Six of the 17 didn't feel any less stressed than those who had eaten burritos. We asked them why.

Their answers put a new spin on our understanding of comfort food.

One said, "When I think of meatloaf, it has brown gravy on top. This one had red, ketchuplike stuff on top." Another said, "When my mom makes meatloaf, she uses a little loaf pan about this size [5x9 inches]. This was made in a huge cafeteria pan."

For these people, it was not only the taste of the meatloaf that mattered. The meatloaf also had to *look* like the meatloaf they had been served when they were growing up. It was both the look and the taste that brought comforting thoughts and feelings to mind.

when they were happy (86 percent) or when they wanted to celebrate or reward themselves (74 percent) than when they were depressed (39 percent), bored (52 percent), or lonely (39 percent). Happy moods = comfort foods. People were almost twice as likely to reach for a comfort food when they were happy than when they were sad.

Moods, however, do seem to influence *what* we choose to eat. People in happy moods tended to prefer healthier foods,

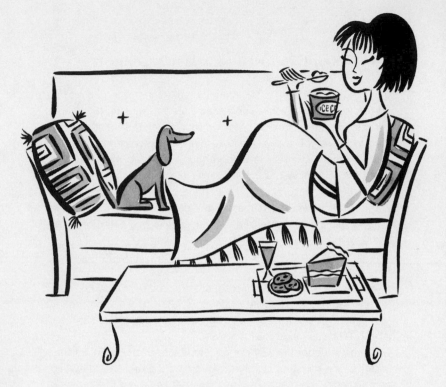

such as pizza or steak. People in sad moods were much more likely to reach for ice cream, cookies, or a bag of potato chips.[2]

Two colleagues, Jeff Inman and Nitika Garg, and I observed this bad mood–bad food bias when we showed people happy movies like *Sweet Home Alabama,* or sad movies like *Love Story.* When we served them hot, buttery popcorn, people ate more when they sobbed along with *Love Story* than when they laughed along with *Sweet Home Alabama.*[3]

We also spent part of one holiday season weighing the uneaten popcorn left behind (or thrown away) after the upbeat movie *My Big Fat Greek Wedding,* and compared it with the popcorn left after the gloomy "intellectual" film *Solaris*. Our garbology detector showed that the average buckets of popcorn left behind in *Solaris* had 29 percent less popcorn in them than those left behind in the happy movie.

I wouldn't want to claim scientific status for these garbological findings, but in combination with survey results, interviews, food diaries, and lab studies, they raise an important comfort-food point. If we want to repair a bad mood, a quick (but temporary) way to do it might be to eat something indulgent that tastes great and gives us that bump of euphoria. It's different when we're in a good mood. If we want to maintain or extend that happy feeling, we can do so by eating a food that scores higher on nutrition and lower on guilt.

The Conditioning of Comfort

Why is macaroni and cheese a comfort food for you, while meatloaf is a comfort food for your brother or sister? Most people can't tell you. Comfort-food connections are almost always subconsciously formed.

To better understand how these connections develop, my lab uses an in-depth interviewing method called "laddering."[4] Laddering is a technique for eliciting the deep connections people have between the characteristics of a food (or product) and their feelings toward it. It's the first tool I teach the researchers in my Lab, and I've taught it to over 1,500 MBA students who have taken my course Understanding Consumer Choice.

A laddering interview is a way to organize a person's free

associations with a food. A psychoanalyst asks a patient on a couch to free associate in order to discover insights and connections that aren't consciously apparent. Laddering serves a similar function, except that instead of searching for the root of a problem, we're searching for the root reason a person became smitten with a particular food.

We start by asking why they like a specific comfort food, and then we keep on asking questions like "Why is that important to you?" or "What do you mean by that?" over and over for about 45 minutes. Everything they say we link with a prior explanation until we have sketched out a crowded, almost unreadable map of all the associations they have with that comfort food. After the interview, we link each key idea with the one mentioned before it and after it. What we end up with is a ladder diagram that starts with very specific associations at the bottom and then gradually works up to the more general goals that the food helps satisfy.

We did comfort-food interviews with 411 adults, who ranged in age from 22 to 78. While there are hundreds of idiosyncratic reasons people articulated for how the foods became comfort foods, two of the more interesting dealt with 1) past associations with the food and 2) personality identification. Here is an example:

Consider Teresa, a woman in her 40s whose favorite comfort food was a bowl of popcorn mixed with a small bag of M&M's. If you asked her why she liked this, she would say that the sweet and salty contrast tasted good. If you asked, "Why is that important to you?" she would say she ends up eating less and feeling less guilty, which makes her feel happy and relaxed. She might also say that it's easy to make, and that it lets her feel domestic "in an odd sort of way." With a little more thought and a little more questioning, we might find that she and her husband (then boyfriend) used to make it in college and it became sort of a personalized or "secret" snack. Eating it brings back college memories and also now seems like a family tradition. Both associations make her feel "cozy and safe." Now, this is really a boiled-down "Cliff's Notes" summary of an intense 45-minute interview. Although all of these connections were in her mind, she wasn't aware of many of them until they emerged during the questioning.

A Mental Map of a Comfort Food: Popcorn Mixed with M&M's

(Read the ladder from the bottom up)

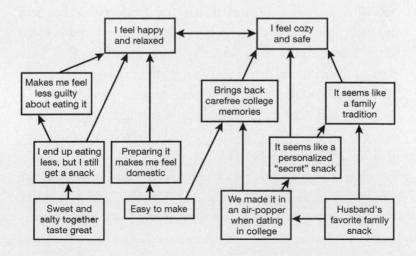

Past associations are the most common reason a food becomes a comfort food. Some of these associations can be linked to specific individuals ("My father loved green bean casserole; we ate it every holiday and on his birthday" or "On Tuesday nights during high school my brother and I used to go to Taco John's and order bean burritos and just talk and laugh about stuff") or specific events ("My mom always gave me soup when it was cold outside or when I was sick and staying home from school"). They're also associated with specific feelings that the person likes to recall or wants to recapture ("We always got ice cream after we won baseball games as a kid" or "I always associate Slurpees with carefree summers"). In some cases, these are vivid iconic experiences we flash on when thinking, tasting, or smelling the food. But even if the memories are vague, the general feelings evoked—feelings of safety, love, homecoming, appreciation, control, victory, or empowerment—are ones that pull us to these foods.

While some people are drawn to a comfort food because of these past associations, others can be drawn toward the same food because they identify with it personally.[5] One person identifies with a type of angel food cake because it is "sweet and petite." Another identifies with soup because it is "warm and nurturing." They begin seeing a food as a comfort food because they subconsciously view it as consistent with their personality.

How do these insights assist us in helping people eat better?

You Are What You Slurp

Does your personality predict your food preferences? I've sat in diners with veteran waitresses who could predict—with surprising accuracy—what a stranger would order when he walked in the door. They could tell by his "look"—how he walked, what he wore, how he looked around.

We wanted to see if there was anything to this. We surveyed 554 soup fanatics and built a statistical personality profile of the type of person most likely to love each of the five most popular soups.[6]

Match the Favorite Soup to the Personality

(Answers on page 151)

1. Chicken Noodle	**A) The Homebody:** Loyal, relaxed stay-at-home who enjoys solitary hobbies (and the occasional talk show).
2. Chili Beef	**B) The Wit:** Sophisticated and intellectual, but a bit sarcastic. Indulges in food, but exercises it off.
3. Vegetable	**C) The Affectionate Reader:** Often a pet owner, and a creative, book-loving thinker.
4. New England Clam Chowder	**D) The Life of the Party:** A competitive, social animal likely to enjoy TV sitcoms like *The Simpsons*.
5. Tomato	**E) The Trendsetter:** Culinary whiz and big dessert lover who is outgoing and adventurous.

When we asked 26 diner waitresses to match these five soups with their five personalities, 21 of the waitresses correctly matched all five. Average score: 83 percent.

The notion of "personality identification" seemed pretty abstract and not very useful when we first came across it in 1996. A couple of years later, the light went on. The soy industry asked our advice on developing and marketing a low-fat meat substitute for nonvegetarians. We soon discovered that personality identification explains why it's harder to get men to eat soy than women. To the strong, traditional, macho, biceps-flexing, all-American male, red meat is a strong, traditional, macho, biceps-flexing, all-American food. Soy is not. To eat it, they would have to give up a food they saw as strong and powerful, like themselves, for a food they saw as weak and wimpy. Soy had two strikes against it before it even got to their plate.[7]

On the other hand, this notion of personality identification might also help explain why it was easier to get some women to gradually switch over to eating more soy foods instead of beef. Some saw soy—largely through their view of tofu—as something soft, delicate, and natural. Just as they saw themselves. Eating it wouldn't be incompatible with their perception of themselves. As a result, soy *didn't* have two strikes against it.

We recommended that if soy producers were to develop food that had been reshaped to look like various cuts of beef, and repackaged and advertised to have more meat-related cues (like pictures of large portions, steak sauce, and barbecuing), it would help men cautiously make the transition. Being realistic, we also recommended that they spend most of their effort on women in their 20s, who can identify with soy and who aren't stuck in 30 years of a cooking rut.

Once you recognize it, personality identification can be found even with foods as mundane as candy bars. A vivid

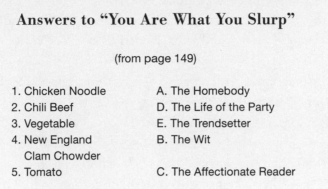

Answers to "You Are What You Slurp"

(from page 149)

1. Chicken Noodle	A. The Homebody
2. Chili Beef	D. The Life of the Party
3. Vegetable	E. The Trendsetter
4. New England Clam Chowder	B. The Wit
5. Tomato	C. The Affectionate Reader

example of personality identification was found in a study of 63 candy bar fanatics. One of the brands we studied was Oh Henry!, a candy bar that tastes a bit like a Snickers bar, but has a much smaller fan club. However, there was a small but mighty group of Oh Henry! lovers who viewed it as a comfort food. In our laddering interviews, we learned that these fanatics viewed it as a "best kept secret" that was unique and stylish in a "think different" sort of way.

A few weeks later, in what they thought was an unrelated survey, these same people were asked to describe themselves. Not ironically, they rated themselves as being unique and stylish in a "think different" sort of way.[8] It wasn't warm, childhood associations that made this candy bar a comfort food, it was the fact that they saw this good-tasting candy bar as unique—just like they saw themselves. Does this mean a more mainstream, follow-the-crowd sort of person wouldn't find Oh Henry! a comfort food? Certainly not. A more mainstream person might be drawn to it for other reasons, perhaps childhood memories. One person who rated himself in this way saw it as a comfort food because his grandfather was named Henry and it happened to be his favorite candy bar.[9]

What about the common assumption that comfort-food preferences are hard-wired during childhood? Our data show this is a myth.

We often found people like Teresa—with her college associations with popcorn and M&M's—who loved comfort foods they had only been introduced to as adults. Sometimes it was a favorite food of their spouses. Other times, it was simply something that was increasingly paired with positive situations.

For example, we found that around one out of eight Chinese graduate students claimed cookies as one of their comfort foods. Cookies aren't common in China or Taiwan. The Chinese diet includes cakelike foods, but even these aren't typically very sweet. Yet within two years of moving to the United States cookies had become a comfort food for some Chinese students.

Here's an example of what we discovered in our interviews. A Taiwanese MBA student arrives in the United States at age 25. She's almost immediately invited to a series of lighthearted business-school receptions where cookies and punch are served—association #1. The next week, her study group takes a break and someone brings out cookies as a snack for everyone—association #2. A couple of weeks later, she goes to a birthday party for a friend, where ice cream is served along with cookies—association #3. As this continues, a subtle connection is made that cookies not only taste good, they're fun. In all these situations, she's been having a good time, and she becomes conditioned to pair cookies with having fun and feeling good.

Eventually when she has a great day and wants to maintain that feeling, she thinks of cookies. On the more discomforting days, when life didn't go her way and she wants to repair her mood, she might also think of cookies.

This is not because her mother was Mrs. Fields. Again, she never tasted a chocolate chip cookie until she was an adult. It's never too late to form new associations to food, and it's never too late for something to become a comfort food.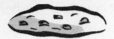

What Are You Really Hungry For?

Do you want a Snickers bar or do you really want a hug? The authors of *Think Thin, Be Thin* offer the following rules of thumb for whether you're responding to physical hunger or feeding a deeper emotional need.[10]

PHYSICAL HUNGER	EMOTIONAL HUNGER
• Builds gradually	• Develops suddenly
• Strikes below the neck (e.g., growling stomach)	• Above the neck (e.g., a "taste" for ice cream)
• Occurs several hours after a meal	• Unrelated to time
• Goes away when full	• Persists despite fullness
• Eating leads to feeling of satisfaction	• Eating leads to guilt and shame

Fifty Years from the Front

What a difference 75 years makes. If popular cookbooks are any indication, most American dinners in the 1930s consisted of either meat and potatoes or potatoes and meat. Chinese food was for the Chinese, Italian food was for Italians, and Mexican food was for Mexicans.

Fast-forward to today. In any town with more than 3,000 people, the best restaurant may well serve Italian food. In that same town, the two restaurants that open the earliest and close the latest may well be the Chinese restaurant on one side of Main Street and the Mexican restaurant on the other.

What happened over the past 50 to 75 years that transformed the way we eat? Mass immigration and explosive industrialization happened. What also happened was World War II.

Being overseas in World War II opened up the culinary world for many American men. French, Italian, and German food tasted pretty good to most returning veterans. They found jobs, started families, and the idea of spaghetti or a bratwurst was not as strange—not as "foreign-sounding"— as it had been five years earlier.

But something was different for the Pacific vets. They returned either loving or hating Chinese food. In interviewing dozens of World War II vets in their homes or in smoky VFW clubs, we discovered that it was easy for the European veteran to learn to appreciate the meat-and-potato-like food of the French, Italians, and Germans. It wasn't radically different from what they were used to. But for the Pacific vet, Chinese food was unlike anything most of them had ever eaten.

So why did some veterans of the South Pacific learn to love Chinese food and others hated it—and still hate it 50 years later? We surveyed 603 World War II veterans from the United States and focused on the 261 who had served with the Army, Navy, or Marine Corps in the South Pacific. During their tour, they would have eaten a number of Chinese-like cuisines. We asked them how often they ate Chinese food and how much they liked it 50 years after the war. We also asked them other questions about their experiences and attitudes.

Forty-six percent of our Pacific veterans enjoyed Chinese food and still ate it with some frequency. But we could find no other characteristics they had in common. Before the war, some had lived in big cities, some on farms. Some had grown up with plenty of food, others had worried about food most of their childhood. Some had graduated from college, others had never seen a ninth-grade classroom. What was the missing link that connected them?

As we later discovered, the answer didn't lie with the people who *liked* Chinese food. It emerged only when we analyzed the data about those soldiers who grew to *hate* Chinese food.

The 31 percent of the Pacific veterans who hated Chinese food were also diverse in terms of where they came from and who they became. Almost all, however, shared one important characteristic. They had experienced frequent and heavy close-quarter combat in the South Pacific. As a result, the local foods they ate there brought up anxious and discomforting feelings—even 50 years later.

In contrast, when we went back to the profiles of those who liked Chinese food, we didn't find any Marines who'd been at Iwo Jima or any infantry soldiers at Guadalcanal. What we found were mechanics, clerks, engineers, and truck drivers—enlisted men who did not experience the war from the front line. Although their wartime experience was a sacrifice, they didn't come home with terrible associations that tainted the taste of food, seemingly forever.[11]

The feelings we have when we first eat a food can follow us for a lifetime. It doesn't matter whether we're an adult or a child. And these insidious, long-gone experiences may even influence the order in which we clean our plate.

Do You Save the Best for Last?

At dinnertime do you eat your favorite foods first or do you tend to save the best for last? The world is divided in half on this issue. We discovered why, but quite accidentally.

The story started when we teamed up with Peter Todd and other behavioral scientists from the Max Planck Institutes in Germany to determine how people evaluate an overall collection of foods (a meal) where the food is uneven (a great appetizer, but a terrible entrée). We thought the answer could provide a key to how our eating patterns have evolved over the past 100 years and might explain why the dinner plate is clean and the salad bowl is not.

Our hypothesis was that when we eat a number of foods in a row our overall evaluation of them will be biased by either the first food or the last. Psychologists refer to this as the power of primacy and recency. That is, our judgment of a meal is biased by our first impression or our last impression. If the middle courses, like the entrée or side dishes, fall short, that should matter less.

If true, this would also be useful knowledge for time-stressed chefs or for the weekend cook who has invited six neighbors over for dinner. If you impress them with your appetizer or dessert, you don't have to worry so much about the food in the middle.

To test this theory, we decided to start with convenient, inexpensive snacks. If it didn't work with snacks, it probably wouldn't work with entrées and appetizers. To find a wide range of snacks that Americans were likely to find either good or bad, we scoured Chicago's Chinatown until my Jeep was filled with unusual treats from China, Korea, Vietnam, Japan, and Thailand. We didn't want familiar brands that would already have strong associations for our eaters, but some of the snacks were types that Americans might like, such as hard candy and fruit-based snacks. Then there were the others, like seaweed candy and blood cake.

We arranged 12 huge bowls of these snacks and invited 183 hungry students in for a late-afternoon "snack buffet." First we asked them to rank-order all 12 snacks from what they thought would be their favorite down to their least favorite. Then we dished up their favorite, their least favorite, and one toward the middle (their sixth favorite). We told them they could have as many snacks as they wanted, but before they could have additional snacks, they had to eat these three. This is when the weeping and the gnashing of teeth began.

Almost everyone reluctantly agreed to continue with the study and to eat the three snacks. After they finished, we asked them to rate their overall experience (on a 1–100 point scale), along with some questions about their background and their childhood. We expected that people who ate their least favorite choice first or last would like the experience less than those who ate it in the middle.

This did not happen. Their ratings appeared almost random. There was nothing interesting—no patterns, no insights. It was a waste of $1,100 of snack food and about 175 of hours of planning, shopping, feeding, cleaning up, and data analysis.

This was nothing new; more than half our studies don't come out as gracefully as we hypothesize.[12] We're used to going back to the drawing board, finding what went wrong, and running the study a different way. This time, however, our return to the drawing board turned up something we had overlooked: almost nobody ate either their favorite food or their least favorite food in the middle. They seemed to use one of two "eating strategies." They either "saved the best for last" or "ate the best one first."

When we looked again at the questionnaires they had completed, we discovered that people who ate the best one first often shared one of two characteristics: they either grew up as a youngest child or came from large families.

The people most likely to save the best for last, on the other hand, had grown up as an only child or as the oldest. They could afford to save their favorite foods as a reward, knowing it would still be waiting for them at the end of the meal. It's different for children in big families, particularly if they're not the oldest. There is competition for food, even when there's plenty to eat. If you don't eat your favorite foods first, you might lose out altogether. Get it while you can.

In the end, our childhood eating habits can follow us for years. If a child becomes conditioned to eat their favorite foods first, they might develop the long-term eating habit of filling up on the high-calorie goodies at the expense of the healthier salads, fruits, and vegetables. That is a recipe for obesity.

Each February, everyone in my Lab volunteers to serve free meals in local soup kitchens, such as the Salvation Army's. Although every person eating there has a different story, one thing they all have in common is that they're hungry. A second thing that many have in common is the order in which they eat their foods and the order in which they get their plates refilled: favorites first. This almost always translates into eating the high-calorie foods first, and the salads, fruits, and vegetables last (if at all).

We have just begun our food-order project, but in combination with our soup kitchen experiences, it's made the people in my Lab uneasy. Once habits are formed, like eating the more caloric food first, how easy are they to change? Let's say that all of the fruits and vegetables in a low-income neighborhood suddenly become fresh and affordable— maybe even free—would that make a difference in what people actually ate? Or would they still fill up on the high-calorie foods?

If a boy grew up not knowing when or what the next meal would be, he would be smart to "eat the best first" any chance he got. The problem with this strategy arises years later when food is more plentiful and he is deciding between a pepperoni pizza or a salad. Being ingrained with fears of food scarcity might mean the pizza disappears without the salad being touched.

Food associations can last for a lifetime. What went on at the dinner table 30 (or even 50) years ago affects us now. We can mindfully override these tendencies, but they still persist when we slip back into mindless eating.

Reengineering Strategy #7: Make Comfort Foods More Comforting

The dieting strategy of saying "I'll never eat fried chicken or ice cream again in my life" is destined for failure. Comfort foods help make life enjoyable. The key is learning how to have your cake and eat it too.

- **Don't deprive yourself.** One reason many diets fail before they even really gain momentum is that they deprive us of the food and lifestyle we enjoy. They also require us to forgo our typical way of life and to focus on calories and on resisting generations of evolution and billions of dollars of food marketing. The best way to begin changing habits is to do so in a way that doesn't make you feel deprived: keep the comfort foods, but eat them in smaller amounts. Our studies also show that most people have at least some comfort foods that are reasonably healthy. Small doses take you a long way.
- **Rewire your comfort foods.** If your comfort foods consist mainly of the four c's—cookies, candies, chips, and cake—all is not lost. Just like the

Chinese graduate student who developed American comfort-food favorites in her 20s, we can rewire our comfort foods. The key is to start pairing healthier foods with positive events. Instead of celebrating a personal victory or smothering a defeat with the "death by chocolate" ice cream sundae, try a smaller bowl of ice cream with fresh strawberries. It's not a big sacrifice, and before long it will start to inch up your "favorites" list.

8

Nutritional Gatekeepers

MOST OF US HAVE the illusion that we're the master and commander of our food choices. As I hope this book has persuaded you by now, we are wrong. Many of these choices are habits. Some we inherited and others were knowingly or unknowingly conditioned by our parents and the food tools they used.

Food tools? Sure. Remember eating your vegetables to get dessert, getting good grades to go to Dairy Queen, cleaning your plate to save all of the starving children in China? A generation later, we are using the same kinds of tools with our children. And as they grow older, they reflect more and more of the inherited and conditioned food habits we have passed down to them like family heirlooms.

If you struggle with your own food heritage, here is where you get your second chance—as a nutritional gatekeeper.

The biggest food influence in our life is the nutritional gatekeeper. This is the person in our home who does most of the food shopping and meal preparation. Regardless of whether they're a great cook or whether they're "culinarily challenged," they have a huge day-by-day influence on their family's nutrition.

The Nutritional Gatekeeper and the Good Cook Next Door

In most households, decisions about what to eat for breakfast, lunch, dinner, and snacks are determined by what foods the grocery shopper—the nutritional gatekeeper—brings into the house. Although they don't always realize it, gatekeepers powerfully shape what food gets eaten both inside and outside the house.

Suppose a teenager wants to eat Pop-Tarts, but there aren't any in the cupboard? The gatekeeper has de facto decided they won't be on the menu. This poor Pop-Tart hungry teenager either has to make a special trip to the grocery store, or pressure Mom or Dad to put them at the top of the next shopping list.

Exactly how much influence does a gatekeeper have?

On a steamy Manila-like August morning in Washington, D.C., in 2005, I met with 800 dieticians, nurses, and physicians at a conference of the American Association of Diabetes Educators. These experts are paid to know how people *should* eat and how they *do* eat. They watch their diabetic patients—and their families—eat day in and day out. I asked them about the nutritional gatekeeper, the person who does most of the shopping and cooking in a household (around 90 percent of the time this is the same person). I asked them to estimate

Fruit Lovers
vs.
Vegetable Lovers

Are fruit lovers different from vegetable lovers? We surveyed 770 people and found some interesting differences:[1]

Compared to the average person, vegetable lovers:

- Like to try new recipes and entertain at home
- Enjoy spicy foods
- Think they cook nutritiously
- Enjoy an occasional glass of red wine with dinner

Compared to the average person, fruit lovers:

- Often eat dessert with dinner
- Spend little time cooking
- Avoid new recipes and entertaining
- Enjoy an occasional candy bar

If we step back, the survey results make sense: fruits are convenient, but veggies often require preparation. Someone who's vegetable-prone may be more accustomed to cooking—and more comfortable with new recipes or the prospect of dinner guests.

Fruits are generally sweeter than vegetables, and fruit lovers may prefer sweeter foods, desserts, and candy. Vegetables, however, run the range from bitter to savory. That's probably why vegetable lovers prefer the strong and savory tastes of exotic or spicy foods, and even the bitter tannins of red wines.

what percentage of the food eaten by these families—snacks, meals, out-of-the-house meals, everything—is controlled by the gatekeeper. Their answers surprised me.

They estimated that the gatekeeper controlled 72 percent of the food decisions of their children and spouse.[2] After all, they were the ones who bought almost everything that was eaten at home, they were the ones who either made their children's lunches or gave them lunch or snack money, and they were the ones who influenced family restaurant orders by what they recommended or ordered themselves.

We have since asked over 2,500 parents to estimate this percentage. Some were 10 points lower or 10 points higher, but the answer was always in the same range. Only one group stood out, because their estimates were consistently high. These were people who also rated themselves as "good

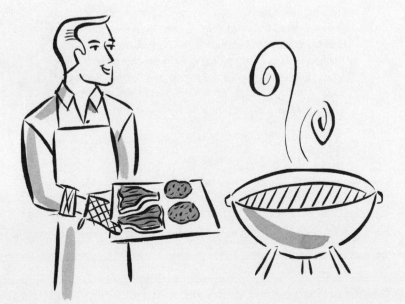

Lessons from the Good Cook Next Door

A study of 317 good cooks showed that most of them tend to fall into one of five basic groups:[3]

- **Giving Cooks (22 percent).** Friendly, well-liked, and enthusiastic, they specialize in comfort foods for family gatherings and large parties. Giving cooks seldom experiment with new dishes, instead relying on traditional favorites. The only fault of the giving cook is that they tend to provide too many home-baked goodies for their family.
- **Healthy Cooks (20 percent).** Optimistic, book-loving, nature enthusiasts who are most likely to experiment with fish and with fresh ingredients, including herbs.
- **Innovative Cooks (19 percent).** The most creative, trend-setting of all cooks. They seldom use recipes; they experiment with ingredients, cuisine styles, and cooking methods.
- **Methodical Cooks (18 percent).** Often weekend hobbyists who are talented, but who rely heavily on recipes. Although somewhat inefficient in the kitchen, their creations always look exactly like the picture in the cookbook.
- **Competitive Cooks (13 percent).** The Iron Chef of the neighborhood. Competitive cooks are dominant personalities who cook in order to impress others. These are perfectionists who are intense in both their cooking and entertaining.

cooks." This made some sense. It was in line with a study we did that showed that many veggie lovers claimed either to be a good cook, to live with a good cook, or to have had a parent who was a good cook.[4] But exactly who were these good cooks, and why were they so influential?

We decided to track down the mysterious North American

Good Cook, take some psychographic snapshots of the species, and decipher their influence. To do this, we surveyed 317 "good cooks" who were considered "above average" by themselves and by at least one other member of their family. They came from a wide range of ethnicities, income levels, and education levels. Besides being good cooks, they all had one thing in common—they had never attended culinary school. Some had learned from a parent, others on their own; some cooked out of necessity, and some for fun. We asked them 152 questions about how they cooked, what they cooked, when they cooked, what kind of person they were, and what they did in their spare time. We found that 82 percent of them fit fairly neatly into one of five personality profiles. We classified them as giving cooks, competitive cooks, healthy cooks, methodical cooks, or innovative cooks.[5]

All of these cooks—except one—appeared to help their families eat healthier. They did this largely through the wide variety of food they served. A varied menu makes eating more pleasurable and can lead family members to expand their tastes beyond the standard fatty, salty, sweet foods for which we have a natural hankering.

Which good cook seemed to have the least positive impact on adult eating habits? Interestingly enough, it was the most common one—the giving cook. Although giving cooks put the stamp of variety on their meals, it was mostly in the form of high-carb entrées, baked goodies, and desserts.

Does this mean that if you're not a good cook, your children are destined to a lifetime of Domino's Pizza and Fritos? No, of course not. One key take-away for us "not so great cooks" is the good we *can* do just by adding more variety to our meals. How? By 1) buying different foods, 2) trying new recipes (including ethnic ones), 3) substituting different ingredients (mainly vegetables and spices) into favorite recipes, 4) taking kids to the grocery store and letting them choose a new, healthy food, or 5) visiting authentic ethnic restaurants. (Sorry, McDonald's is not a Scottish restaurant.)

When a child develops a taste for a wide range of foods, healthy foods can be more easily substituted for less healthy ones.[6] He or she may even discover favorites other than pizza, French fries, and Juicy Juice. Will your daughter learn to *love* broccoli? Maybe not, but she'll probably be more willing to eat it occasionally for dinner or with a low-calorie ranch dressing as a snack.[7]

Food Inheritance:
Like Mother, Like Daughter

We sometimes hear that a child "inherited" his sweet tooth, or her love for vegetables or spicy foods, from a parent. Although the genetics jury is still out, it's clear that children adopt some of their mother's tastes when they're still snoozing away in the womb. Remember that pregnant women

The Baby Buffet

Most children go through a finicky eating stage at two years of age, but when they are one year old, anything within arm's-length goes into their mouths. This provides a great opportunity to introduce them to all sorts of healthy new tastes—even non-kidlike vegetables.

My Lab recently began what we call "Operation Baby Buffet." We enlisted a nationwide panel of parents of one-year-old children, and we instructed them (under the guidance of a pediatrician) to be adventurous—even bold—in the variety of foods they put in front of their grabby baby or which they blend into baby food (including—starting with the letter "A"—avocados, asparagus, and fresh anchovies).

Our hypothesis is that all of this variety will predispose their little taste buds to liking a wide range of healthy foods. Although this predisposition may go dormant for a few years, it might awaken down the road when they mysteriously find themselves hungry for Camembert cheese and gingered beets with raisins.[8]

who drank carrot juice in their last trimester significantly increased how much their children preferred carrot-flavored cereal months later.[9]

Not only do they develop prenatal munchie preferences, children also start learning what they like and *don't* like before they're four months old. They do this by picking up on signals a parent or caretaker unconsciously gives about whether a food is tasty or not.

This was first discovered in the Massachusetts Reformatory for Women during the 1940s. The women incarcerated there were able to keep their children under three years of age and to frequently visit them and their caretakers in the nursery. Records were kept on what the children ate, so it was noticed when their juice preferences abruptly changed. The psychologist at the reformatory, Sibylle Escalona, began to suspect that the caretakers were unconsciously influencing what the children preferred.[10]

Her report starts out, "It came to attention accidentally that many of the babies under four months of age showed a consistent dislike for either orange or tomato juice." She then went on to report that babies who had refused to drink orange juice for about three weeks would all of a sudden turn into orange-juice lovers within two or three days. She traced these abrupt shifts to changes in caretakers. Upon being interviewed, it was found that a couple of the new caretakers had a strong preference for orange juice and a dislike for tomato juice. Somehow this was passed along to the infants.

But how? Interestingly, even two-day-old babies are known to be able to imitate facial expressions of adults.[11] It could be that these caretakers subconsciously showed subtle signs of acceptance or rejection based on what they personally felt toward the foods. A fleeting smile or grimace might go a long way toward explaining why one baby has Daddy's sweet tooth and another has Mommy's love for vegetables. It also makes good sense that people feeding babies pretend to taste the food (Mmm . . . yummy!") and open their mouths and play "airplane hangar" when feeding the little tykes.[12]

Escalona's accidental discovery has aged well. Watching someone grimace when eating scares elementary children

away from even an otherwise tasty food.[13] Smiles and friend-
liness work in reverse—you can attract more children to
new foods with honey than with vinegar. When a friendly
adult repeatedly gave children either canned unsweetened
pineapple or cashews, they quickly learned to like the new
food more than when it was given to them by a less friendly
adult.[14]

It is not only our tastes that our children can inherit. It
also can be our attitudes about food and eating. In one Yale
study of normal-weight one-year-olds, mothers who were
highly preoccupied with weight issues were more likely to
be erratic in their behavior during meals. Sometimes they
urged their one-year-olds to eat more, sometimes to eat less,
and sometimes they rushed their feedings. They were also
much more emotionally aroused when feeding their babies
compared to mothers who weren't concerned with weight
issues.[15] Children see this anxiety and these food obsessions
at a tender *tabula rasa* age.

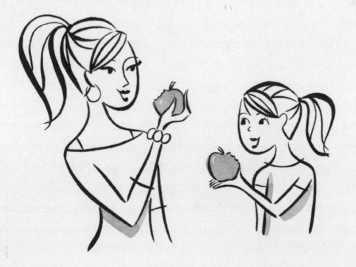

Is It Baby Fat or Real Fat?

The answer partly depends on the parents. A study of 854 Washington State children under three years old showed that a child is nearly three times as likely to grow up obese if one of his parents is obese. If you're overweight, your child has a 65–75 percent chance of growing up to be overweight.[16]

So, is that little paunch on your fourth grader baby fat?

Not if you're sporting the same paunch.

Food Conditioning and the Popeye Project

In turn-of-the-century pre-Bolshevik Russia, physiologist Ivan Pavlov rang a bell and fed his dogs frequently enough for them to associate the ringing of the bell with food. Eventually the dogs started to salivate every time they heard the bell—even if there was no food.

Eighty years later, psychologist Leann Birch reran Pavlov's classic experiment, with a few twists. She and her team repeatedly gave preschool children snacks in a specific location where they would always see a rotating light and hear a certain song. They came to associate the light and the song with snack time and eating. One day, shortly after they had finished lunch, she turned on the light and played the song. Doggone it, they started eating again.[17]

But we don't need lights and music to condition our children. We can powerfully do so with our words and behavior.

Take the Popeye project.[18] My Lab is trying to understand

why some children develop powerfully positive associations with healthy foods—such as broiled fish, broccoli, and even seaweed—that are not typically liked by most children. In beginning this work, we conducted separate interviews with children and with their parents. These interviews took an abrupt right turn a couple of weeks after they began.

We expected that the children with positive associations toward healthy foods had "inherited" them from their parents in the ways I've already discussed. While true in many cases, in other cases, the parents didn't leave this to chance. These parents explicitly associated the foods with a positive benefit—such as "spinach makes you strong like Popeye." Some children grew up learning to love fish because their parents told them it would make them smart. Others were told to eat carrots so they could see far distances, bananas so they would have strong bones, and fruit so they could keep cool in the summer. A couple of children (whose parents were originally from China) even grew up eating—and loving—seaweed because they were told it would prevent "stomach sickness" (or, as their parents later clarified, goiters.)[19] Hard to see that one as a big motivator to a four-year-old. The first day of school would be one to remember: "Hi, I'm Jennifer. What I did on my summer vacation was go to the beach and eat seaweed so I can be goiter-free."

We've interviewed a couple hundred three- to five-year-olds in the Popeye Project so far, and we've collected a lot of insights related to healthy eating—and some surprises. At one day-care center outside of Syracuse, New York, a number of the children had uncharacteristically strong preferences for broccoli. This caught our attention because this bitter vegetable is not as kid-friendly as others (such as carrots and

peas). Many of the children told us they loved broccoli because their friends liked it or because it was "cool." Most of
these associations we could trace back to two little brothers.
In their laddering interviews both said broccoli reminded
them of dinosaur trees, and they liked it because of that.
This didn't make much sense, but because of the far-reaching
impact it seemed to have on the rest of the day-care group,
we interviewed their mother in person. We discovered she
had convinced them that broccoli looked like a
dinosaur tree and when they ate broccoli, they
could pretend they were "long-necked dinosaurs
eating the dinosaur trees." At the dinosaur-
loving age of three and five, that was pretty cool,
and it quickly became pretty cool to their friends.
Brainwashing, conditioning, or just a smart
parent? *Viva la brontosaurus!*

My Lab tried to leverage this with a vacation Bible
School group a short time ago. The children could choose
what they wanted from a lunch buffet, but each day we
would rename foods to give them better associations. For instance, when we renamed peas "power peas," the number of
children taking them nearly doubled. The most embarrass-
ing poetic license we took was with a V8-like vegetable juice.
We ran out of it on the days we renamed it "Rainforest
Smoothie."

These associations can also work the other way around.
Negative associations can be made with unhealthy foods.
While there aren't too many published studies on this, it's
an area rich with anecdotes.

Joyce is an interesting example. When I knew her as an
adult, she never had cravings for cake and cookies. For 45

Time-Honored Strategies for Dodging Vegetables

Today's kids stick to the same classic vegetable-avoidance strategies as their parents used. According to a 1999 Market Facts, Inc.,
study conducted for Green Giant, the three top strategies are:[20]

40%—Push vegetables around on plate so it looks like
there's less
16%—Feed them to the dog
12%—Give them to a younger sibling or to a vegetable
lover

years, she's never had to fight the gravitational pull that
these sweet snacks have on most of us. Why no apparent
sweet tooth? It's almost a *Manchurian Candidate* brainwashing explanation. As a little girl, her mother repeatedly
told her that eating sweet snacks between meals was what
low-class people did.[21] Extreme, yes. Politically incorrect, yes.
Yet because there were no sweet snacks available and because
they had an (unmerited) stigma attached to them, Joyce never
developed the taste for these foods that bedevils many of us.

Setting Serving-Size Habits for Life

A fat-forming transformation in our eating habits takes
place between the ages of three and five. You can give three-
year-olds a lot of food, and they will simply eat until they are

no longer hungry. They are unaffected by serving size. By age five, however, they will pretty much eat whatever they're given. If they are given a lot, they'll eat a lot, and it will even influence their bite size.

The Four Unhealthy Food-Tool Extremes

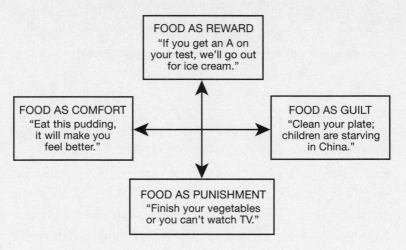

This has been vividly shown by Leann Birch at Penn State and Jennifer Fisher at the Baylor Medical School.[22] When they gave three- or five-year-old children either medium-size or large-size servings of macaroni and cheese, the three-year-olds ate the same amount regardless of what they were given. They ate until they were full, and then they stopped. The five-year-olds rose to the occasion and ate 26 percent more when given bigger servings. Almost exactly the same thing happens to adults. We let the size of a serving influence how much we eat.

Serving size is a problem at mealtime, but it's also a big

problem at snack time. What is a healthy-size snack? Children tend to think that a serving size is open-ended and up for negotiation—it is pretty much whatever food is available and whatever they can weasel out of their parents. If a candy bar comes in a two-ounce package, two ounces must be the correct serving. If the candy bar comes in a four-ounce package, four ounces must be the correct serving.

Suppose you make a peanut butter and jelly sandwich as a snack and give your child half of it. Is the serving size half the sandwich? Not if the other half of the sandwich is still sitting on the counter. At that point, a serving includes anything that's left that can be eaten. What happens if you buy raisins in bulk and give your child a quarter cup of them? If the big container is visible, you may face a campaign for more.

How do we adjust serving size to be more reasonable and less negotiable?

If you buy in bulk to save money, you can use the Baggie trick. Remember that none of us really seem to know the amount of a "correct" serving size. We typically look at whatever is wrapped or served and we assume that must be one serving. We can use this notion with our children by giving them their snacks not on a plate, but by putting them in a Baggie (or even in a small Tupperware container).

Like adults, children use external cues to determine whether they want more to eat. If they think more is available, they can easily think they're still hungry. For instance, in one of our pilot studies, we gave five-year-olds at a day-care center six mini-size cookies in either a Ziploc bag or on a plate. After they finished the cookies, we asked them if they thought there were any more. Children who were given cookies on a plate believed that there were more left in the

The "Half-Plate Rule" of Balanced Meals

What is a balanced meal? Here's an easy rule of thumb for meal planning. For lunch and dinner, half the plate should be vegetables and fruits and the other half should be protein and starch. There are variations on this theme (such as the Idaho Plate Method),[23] but if you remember this basic Half-Plate Rule, you won't think that spaghetti and meatballs is a balanced meal (add a salad).

kitchen—and they wanted them. Children who had been given Baggies were more likely to believe that the cookies were all gone and that snack time was over.

Reengineering Strategy #8:
Crown Yourself as the Official Gatekeeper

For better or worse, the nutritional gatekeeper controls around 72 percent of what your family eats. Children eat what tastes good and what's convenient and what portion size they see as appropriate. You can use this to help create positive lifetime food patterns.

- **Be a good marketer.** Foods should be neither a punishment nor a reward. Healthy foods can, however, be fresh, crunchy, refreshing, and make you strong, smart, and maybe even "goiter-free." (They might even be what long-necked dinosaurs ate.) Be convincing.

- **Offer variety.** Some of our early findings suggest that the more foods you expose your child to, the more nutritionally well-rounded he or she will become. Trying new recipes, new ingredients, ethnic foods, and different types of restaurants will all help mix it up and break the junk-food habit.
- **Use the Half-Plate Rule.** Around the house, the Half-Plate Rule can lead to more-balanced meals, and it can give your children the basic pattern for a healthy meal. Is steak and potatoes a balanced meal? No, it's only half of the plate—you still need a vegetable or salad for the other half.
- **Make serving sizes official.** Provide "official" servings by giving your children their snacks in sealed Baggies, in Tupperware, or in Saran Wrap. Don't let them see extra snacks. We found that any extra snacks on the counter increase the amount they see as a serving size. Clear off the counter at snack time.

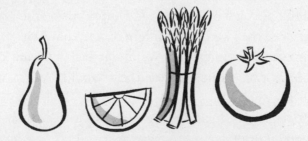

9

Fast-Food Fever

WHY IS FAST FOOD conquering the world? For one, because we have been genetically designed to love it. More accurately, it has been designed to love *us,* by giving us the tastes that generations of evolution have caused us to crave. We are hardwired to love the taste of fat, salt, and sugar. Fatty foods gave our ancestors the calorie reserves to weather food shortages. Salt helped them retain water and avoid dehydration. Sugar helped them distinguish sweet edible berries from the sour poisonous ones. Through our taste for fat, salt, and sugar, we learned to prefer the foods that were most likely to keep us alive.

Almost everything we love about fast food are things that our hunter-gatherer forefathers would, well, kill for. French fries and chips have salt and fat, donuts and Pop-Tarts have fat and sugar, Coke and Pepsi have sugar and salt, and candy bars pretty much have them all.

Some see this as an Us vs. Them world. They believe that fast food is addictive, a conspiracy to destroy our health. They believe that manipulative companies fill fast food with fat, salt, and sugar because they know we will eat it, love it, and come back again and again. Do food companies put ingredients in their food that they know we will eat and love? Absolutely—they are guilty as charged. So is your grandmother, who added mysterious spices (like too much salt) to her secret pasta sauce, loaded her cookies with butter and sugar, and basted the Thanksgiving turkey with its own fat—its own fat! She is guilty as charged.

But your grandmother is no more guilty than we are when we have friends over and add all the spices, butter, and sugar we can to the dinner so that our friends will say, "Hey, that was great." And she is no more guilty than many high-end chefs. In their reservations-only restaurants, taste reigns supreme. Some signature dishes at popular expense-account restaurants contain whole sticks of butter. These are dishes to die for.

Fast-food companies give us the taste we want, and they top it off with two more key attractions: good value and maximum convenience. There's no need to defrost the hamburger at noon or for Grandmother to slave over a hot stove when you can say, "Value Meal #2—large," without leaving your car.

We need to keep in mind that the typical person pulling in to a fast-food parking lot is not driving a BMW or Range Rover that they bought with cash, and they're not eating on an expense account. The typical person is more likely to "have a couple of bucks in his pocket and is looking to get as much good food for that money as he can," according to Eric Haviland, Director of Strategy for

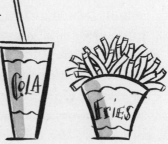

Taco John's.[1] Consistent with this, Taco John's rival, Taco Bell, abandoned its low-calorie Border Light menu in the mid-1990s. Ten years later, their positioning statement is "Feel Full." For a hungry person with a couple bucks in his pocket for lunch, feeling full is a whole lot more tempting than nibbling on a salad with vinaigrette on the side. The people most critical of fast food are usually not those in the "couple of bucks in their pocket" market segment.[2]

The Variety and Convenience of Having It Our Way

Along with giving us the taste for fat, sugar, and salt, our caveman genetics led us to prefer variety in our diet. The more types of foods we ate, the more likely we were to get the wide range of nutrients we needed. We didn't have to know the difference between vitamin C, riboflavin, and a complex carbohydrate. Our natural inclination for variety made sure we got enough of each. And if the food was convenient, all the better.

Remember what happened to the hungry rat in Chapter 4 when it smelled the scent of a killer hawk? Like the rat, the less time our ancestors had to spend strolling around looking for food, the less likely they were to meet something bigger and hungrier than they were. Convenience actually had survival value for them.

Because of this desire to follow the path of least effort, we get convenient easy-to-open packaging, vending machines on every floor, and fast-food restaurants at convenient corners. We also get the chance to buy almost any ready-to-eat or heat-and-serve food we want. And if warming up the food is too inconvenient, we also get drive-throughs and free pizza delivery.

The Magnificent Seven—The Most Commonly Ordered Restaurant Foods[3]

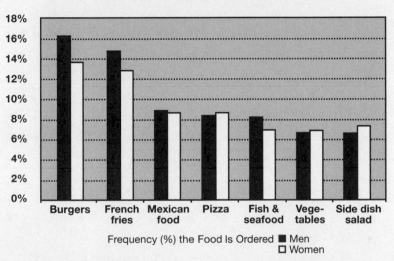

Frequency (%) the Food Is Ordered ■ Men
□ Women

We want variety, convenience, and value, and we get it. Your sandwich wrapper at Subway advertises that it has a variety of seven sandwiches with six grams of fat or less. Your sandwich wrapper at Burger King also has information printed on it. It says, "You have the right to have things your way. You have the right to scarf, wolf, or hork down this hamburger. You have the right to eat it like a dainty little bird. You have the right to order another. You have the right to it being as good as the first one." I don't know how you "hork" down a hamburger, but I'm sure it's a constitutional freedom.

What has increasingly come under fire, however, is not what fast-food restaurants print on their posters and tray liners. It's what they have left off—nutrition information.

The McSubway Study and Information Illusions

Someone somewhere came up with the notion that if we could get everyone in the world to pass a nutrition quiz, we would all eat our fruits and vegetables and live trimly and happily ever after. Most of us know fruit and vegetables are good for us, but we file this information under "Things We Know and Choose to Ignore." For some of us, this is a pretty huge file:

- We know we're supposed to do our sit-ups every morning. Most of us do exactly one; the one it takes to get out of bed.
- We know we're supposed to change our oil every 3,000 miles. Yet some of us wait until the day the window-sticker reminder turns yellow, falls off, and sticks to our shoe when we get out of the car.
- We know we're supposed to floss after every meal. I don't think even dentists do it that often.

Despite our tendency to ignore inconvenient truths, many well-meaning people are campaigning hard to have detailed nutrition information attached to every piece of food within reach. In that world, the king of nutrition information is the Subway restaurant chain.

Subway is all about information. They have nutrition information on posters, napkins, cups, tray liners, and buttons. Even their ads talk about nutrition and fresh ingredients, or they talk about Jared (the star of their commercials), or they talk about Jared talking about nutrition and fresh ingredients. So if Subway is the good king in our kingdom of Eat-a-Lot, who is the villain?

Some say it's none other than Ronald McDonald. After all, even as Subway was putting their heart, soul, and fat content on every piece of paper in the restaurant, McDonald's hid theirs in tiny type on a poster that couldn't be read because it was too close to the heat from the fry vat. Just supersize me, and forget about it.

In 2003, a Food Forum hearing was held at the Institute of Medicine of the National Academies in Washington, D.C.[4] At this closed hearing, one of the presenters held Subway up as the icon of responsibility and consumer education. After the presentation, someone—okay, it was me—had the audacity to ask, "When people eat at Subway, they are surrounded with information. Do you have any data on whether they pay attention to it, or whether it influences how much they eat?" You would have thought we were in

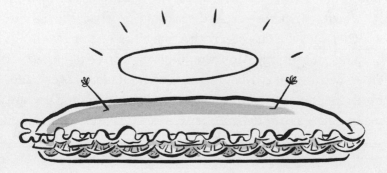

some medieval castle and I had just announced that the world might not be flat. There was silence and then righteous head-shaking and snickering. The speaker said, "But of course," in a patronizing, you-silly-child sort of way. "Of course people read it and of course they eat healthier because of it."

Of course, there was no pesky evidence to support this assertion. Nor was there any data that people eat healthier because of the information. They didn't even have evidence that anybody read or remembered the nutrition facts by the time they finished their lunch.

When you go to a "healthy" restaurant, do you pay attention to what you eat, or do you eat with abandon because you think it's generally healthy? Maybe you even order a cookie to congratulate yourself on your healthy meal? What we did to answer these questions would eventually come to be known as the McSubway Study.[5]

My French colleague Pierre Chandon and I, along with a team of undergraduates, interviewed a total of 250 people right after they finished lunch at various Subway locations. We asked them how many total calories they thought they'd eaten, what specific nutrition information they remembered reading in the restaurant, and whether the information would influence them in the future. We also asked them to list exactly what they ate—the sandwich, what it had on it, whether they ate chips, whether they had one or two refills of soda, everything. After the interviews were done, we sat down with the nutritional posters and calculated every calorie they ordered and ate. This way we could compare how many calories they *thought* they'd eaten with how many they *actually* ate.

Then we did exactly the same thing at McDonald's restaurants that were located within 150 feet of these Subway restaurants.

Of the 250 people leaving McDonald's, only 57 were even remotely able to recount any nutritional information about the food they just ate. While 18 of them recalled that McDonald's was offering some lower-calorie options such as salads or low-fat wraps, only five of them had ordered one. The most recounted nutritional take-away was that the food was caloric and not healthy, quickly followed by "but it tastes great." When asked if more nutrition information would change what they ate, they pretty much said, "Probably not." The average McLuncher ate and drank a whopping 1,093 calories, but they estimated they ate only 876. That's 25 percent more than they thought.

Of the 250 people leaving Subway, 157 recalled some form of nutrition information and 63 of them correctly recalled that a number of sandwiches had under 6 grams of fat. The rest had a general impression that the food was "healthy," but said they did not pay any attention to the specifics. This "health halo" led many of these people to infer all Subway food was less caloric than is the case. Two even believed that the sandwiches had less than seven calories apiece.

What about how much they ate? Most of the 157 people who recalled nutritional information from Subway ignored the low-fat sandwiches and stampeded straight to the high-calorie ones with meatballs, cold cuts, and bacon. And most of them did not hold the mayo and cheese—77 percent ate their sandwich with cheese and 79 percent with some sort of sauce, 53 percent ordered and finished a bag of potato chips, and 27 percent couldn't resist the chunky cookies by the cash register. Oh, and the drinks: 37 percent ordered soft drinks with calories, and 41 percent headed back for at least one refill.

The average Sub-diner thought he or she was eating 495 calories, but instead ate 677—34 percent more than he or she thought.

Those eating at Subway ate under the illusion that everything they touched was good for them. Those eating at McDonald's seemed to have a less rose-tinted view. McDonald's ads never claimed that french fries and double bacon cheeseburgers make you skinny.

Subway's different. If people don't infer nutrition and weight-loss from the napkins, tray liners, and cups, they think they remember it from the ads. It seems to give them false confidence in what they are eating, and it gives a health halo to all the Subway foods, including the mayonnaise, bacon, potato chips, cookies, and large drinks.

Still, the Subway diners remembered more and ate less than those at McDonald's. And times they are a-changing at Mickey D's. Not only did 2006 bring us nutrition info on McWrappers, it also brought us a leaner Ronald McDonald, who seems to have swapped a few french fries for exercise. Let's watch for him next year in the Iron Man Triathlon.

Do Low-Fat Labels Make Us Fat?

This is a world of fat-free, carb-free, and sugar-free products. When we see these labels, we tend to assume the food

The "10–20" Rule and the Ice Water Diet

In every beverage study we conduct, people underestimate the calories they drink—usually by about 30 percent. It doesn't matter whether it's soft drinks, milk, juice, or wine, although fountain machines pose the biggest danger.

My Lab developed a "10–20" rule of thumb for teaching people to estimate the number of calories in a drink. "Thin drinks" (like soft drinks, punch, juice, and milk) are about 10 calories per ounce and "thick drinks" (smoothies and meal replacement shakes) are about 20 calories per ounce. It's ballpark, but it's better than mindless drinking. Just poured a 32-ounce Coke at McDonald's? Think 320 calories, including ice.

Interestingly, if you load that drink with ice, you'll actually burn off a few of those calories. Since your body has to use energy to heat up an iced beverage, you actually burn about one calorie for every ice-cold ounce you drink.[6] So that 32-ounce drink will take you 35 calories to warm up.

No big deal? If you drink the recommended eight 8-ounce glasses of water a day, and if you fill those 64 ounces with ice, you'll burn an extra 70 calories a day. *That's* approaching the mindless margin.

---

is good for us. In our black-and-white view, most food is good or not good. But does low-fat automatically equal "healthy"?

When Nabisco came out with the SnackWell's line of fat-free cookies, they flew off the shelves, partly because there were at least some people who believed they could eat them until they became supermodels. After six months and six pounds, if these brand champions had bothered to take a magnifying glass to the label, they would've found that these cookies were loaded with sugar and had only about 30 percent fewer calories than standard brands. The same applies to many fat-free and reduced-fat products. Often the reduced-fat version isn't much lower-calorie than the regular version. Yet because we can tend to view foods as black or white, we can always fall into the trap of thinking something is either 100 percent healthy or that it's not.

The flashing red light of the McSubway Study warns us that we can easily let our general impression of a food mislead us. Think you are safe as long as you stay away from fast food and stick to a lunch of tofu and low-fat granola? If so, you have just run another light.

Take granola. Whereas low-fat granola is indeed lower in fat than regular granola, it's only about 10 percent lower in calories.[7] It doesn't take a lot of mindless, guilt-free eating to scarf down an extra 10 percent of granola while thinking you're "doing your body good."

In one segment of the *Hazzard County* video-watching

Fat Matters, but Calories Count

	REGULAR VERSION	REDUCED-FAT VERSION
Fig Cookies (1 cookie)	56 calories	51 calories
Chocolate Chip Cookies (3 cookies)	160 calories	150 calories
Peanut Butter (2 Tbsp)	191 calories	187 calories
Vanilla Frozen Yogurt (1 cup)	104 calories	100 calories
Chicken Noodle Soup (1 cup)	120 calories	140 calories
Granola (1 serving)	196 calories	173 calories

study, Pierre Chandin and I gave out bags of granola labeled either "Low-Fat Rocky Mountain Granola" or "Regular Rocky Mountain Granola." In reality, all the granola was low-fat. While people watched the video, they munched on the granola, but those given the granola labeled "low-fat" kept munching long after the other group stopped. And when we weighed the remains after the movie, those eating what they thought was low-fat ate 49 percent more. Even though all the granola was low-fat, this translated into 84 more calories.

Everyone is tricked by low-fat labels. But, in a cruel twist, they have an even more dramatic impact on those who are overweight. For instance, when we offered one study group low-fat chocolate, the overweight people loaded up on 89 more calories—46 percent more than when it had a regular label. While regular-weight people also got fooled by low-fat halos, their common sense prevailed—they ate only 16 percent more.[8]

If we're looking for an excuse to eat, low-fat labels give it to us.

Health Halos and Nutrition Labels

Labels can also mislead us because we sometimes read things into them that aren't true.[9] Don't believe it? Here's a case in point.

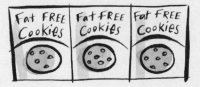

Supersized Diet-Size

Even diet foods have supersized. Lean Cuisine has come up with a
frozen dinner with 100 bonus calories, called "Hearty Portions," and
Weight Watchers has introduced Smart Ones, with larger portion
sizes than their regular fare.

As shoppers turned the corner of aisle 2 in a small
neighborhood grocery store 120 miles south of Chicago,
they were greeted with free samples of two types of nutrition bars—one with health claims and one without.

Actually the nutrition bars were exactly the same, only
the labels were different. Both were in yellow packages with
black letters, but some claimed that the nutrition bar contained soy and helped reduce the risk of heart disease.

After the customers were given the bars with the health
labels, they not only believed that the bars helped reduce
the risk of heart disease, but they also believed they helped
reduce the risk of other diseases (including diabetes and
cancer). Some even reported the bar would reverse damage
that had been caused by other foods—an antidote to junk
food. One little health claim gave the bar an instant halo,
making people believe that the entire bar was much healthier than it was.[10]

Okay, so this wasn't the PowerBar company testing different packaging ideas, it was my Lab. And we weren't interested in soy, per se, we were interested in the health halos

that people give to functional foods in general. (Functional foods are those that provide health benefits beyond their nutritional value.)[11]

What we found shows one danger of health claims on labels. True, people believed the nutrition bar was healthier, but they tended to go too far. Along with believing it would counteract junk food, some even said it would probably reduce the risk of birth defects.

We typically don't want to spend much time reading labels or thinking about them.[12] Instead, we come up with a general idea about whether the product is good for us, and everything follows from that. Soy is good for us, so this soy bar must have all sorts of magical, curative properties.[13]

The same goes for many popular "health cues." If a sandwich has the "heart healthy" sign on it and says it has six grams of fat, we probably know that doesn't include mayo, oil and vinegar, double cheese, potato chips, and a drink. We may know it, but we want to forget it. We want to say, "Looks healthy to me," so we can pile on the rest. In this way, we end up overeating what we think is healthy. Regardless of the serving size.

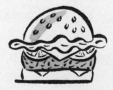

What Serving Size?

Do people pay attention to serving sizes? No. Not under normal circumstances. Like most information on a label, it's ignored by most people. If one serving of Cheetos is 28 grams, who knows how much that is? When we're faced with a big, multi-serving bag or box, a serving is pretty much whatever we eat in one sitting.

Serving sizes start to make sense only when foods are individually packaged. A vending machine–size bag of M&M's (about 57 of them) is one serving to most of us. If we're instead given one of those little Halloween-size bags of M&M's (about 28 of them), that is one serving. The label on a 20-ounce bottle of Coke says it's 2.5 servings, but how many of us plan to split it with the stranger next to us? Maybe we're just 2.5 times the size of the people who make these labels.

The size of a bag or a bottle tells us what we think a serving size should be. Here's a case in point: When we were doing our granola studies, Pierre Chandon and I also tested the effect of serving-size labels on consumption. We gave some of our moviegoers regular granola in bags labeled one serving, others were given bags labeled two servings, and a third group were given bags that had no serving-size information. All of these bags were the same size—640 calories.

This serving-size information was impossible for them to miss. Unlike normal packaging, it was in a large typeface and one of few things on the label, and in this case it had an effect. The more servings the people thought were in the bag, the less they ate. If they thought the bag contained one serving, they ate 207 calories. If they thought it contained two servings, they ate 39 percent less.

If the bag had no serving-size marking on it, how many servings do you think the typical person estimated was inside? Even though it was filled with 640 calories of granola, people assumed it was one serving.

The bottom line: Six 100-calorie servings in separate bags is six servings. Empty them all out into one big 600-

Decoding Labels and Health Claims

Haven't yet cracked the Da Vinci Code the FDA developed for product labels? Here Is a guide:

Low—The product doesn't have a lot of a particular substance, but it still has enough to make a difference in your diet. For example, "low calorie" means 40 calories or less per serving; "low fat" means three grams or less of total fat.

Reduced—A nutritionally altered product—such as reduced fat— contains at least 25 percent less fat than the "regular version."

Less—Has the same meaning as "reduced," but a food might not be altered nutritionally.

Light or Lite—A nutritionally altered product that contains a third fewer calories or half the fat or sodium of the original food.

Free—A product that has virtually no fat, saturated fat, calories, sugars, sodium, or cholesterol. "Virtually" means a trace amount may remain.

Lean and Extra-Lean—These terms refer to meat. "Lean" means one serving has less than 10 grams of total fat, 4.5 grams of saturated fat, and 95 milligrams of cholesterol. "Extra-lean" means one serving has less than 5 grams of total fat, 2 grams of saturated fat, and 95 milligrams of cholesterol.

calorie bowl, and one serving is now however much we want to eat.

De-Marketing Obesity and De-Supersizing

All food companies are the same in two respects. It doesn't matter whether you see them as junk-food sinners or health-food saints. It doesn't matter whether they manufacture Twinkies on a mile-long production line or hand-form organic soy burgers to sell in the Williams-Sonoma catalog.

They all have this in common: First, they don't care if you eat the food, as long as you repeatedly buy it. Second, they want to make a profit. Maybe in the other order.

This is important to understand, because some people believe that McDonald's, or Kraft, or Häagen-Dazs are in business to make us fat. In reality, McDonald's could care less whether we buy a large combo meal, eat half, and then throw the other half away. What they care about is that we buy it from them and not from Hardee's, Wendy's, or Jack in the Box. They make their money when they sell something. They aren't interested in what happens after we shuffle over to the McTable with our tray. The same would have been true of my Uncle Lester, the corn farmer. If you'd told him, "I want to buy three dozen ears of sweet corn, take them home, leave them in the refrigerator for a month, and then throw them out," he would have sold them to you.

Companies want to make a profit. If, starting tomorrow at noon, we all went into Taco Bell and Burger King and ordered only salads, their menus would change faster than you could say "Lite Italian." Within a year, people would be able to eat at a Taco Salad Bell anytime they wanted to make a run for the border. Within another year there would be a Broccoli King.

Recent surveys of all foods ordered in restaurants show that burgers, French fries, pizza, and Mexican food comprise almost 50 percent of *all* food purchases. We order these foods *five* times more frequently than we order vegetables or side salads.[14] Burger King offers a side salad that costs less than medium fries. But as my local Burger King manager told me, the fries win out about 30 to 1. It's the burgers and fries that keep people coming back.

Fast-food companies don't care what we decide to eat for lunch. They do care, however, about their corporate image, and they listen to customer demand. When McDonald's realized how many vegetarians there were, Veggie Burgers made it onto the menu. When the low-carb diet club grew in membership, low-carb burgers appeared at Burger King. As Burger King has said for many years, "Have It Your Way." Each tray liner at Burger King used to house its own Bill of Rights. Would the Founding Fathers roll their eyes? Absolutely. Deny us this particular pursuit of happiness? Absolutely not.

No food company is in business to make us fat, they're in business to sell us food. If we want fattening food to mindlessly eat, companies will fix it. But they will also fix us healthy food that we can mindfully eat if they can profitably do so. In fact, most of the leading packaged-goods companies—like General Mills and Kraft—are experimenting with new ideas, programs, and

Having It Your Way
The Burger King Bill of Rights

You have the right to have things your way.
You have the right to hold the pickles and hold the lettuce.
You have the right to mix Coke and Sprite.
You have the right to a Whopper sandwich with extra tomato, extra onion, and triple cheese.
You have the right to have that big meal, sleepy feeling when you're finished.
You have the right to put a paper crown on your head and pretend you're ruler of "your make-believe kingdom here."
You have the right to have your chicken fire-grilled or fried.
You have the right to dip your fries in ketchup, mayonnaise, BBQ sauce, or mustard.
Or not.
You have the right to laugh until soda explodes from your nose.
You have the right to stand up and fight for what you believe in.
You have the right to sit down and do nothing.
You have the right to eat a hot and juicy fire-grilled burger prepared just the way you like.
You have the right to crumple this Bill of Rights into a ball and shoot hoops with it.
Have It Your Way.

products that they think will provide win-win solutions for them and their consumers. Using some of our mindless eating principles, let's look at what a sharp, nutrition-conscious marketer could do to profitably offer us food that can help us eat more mindfully. Let's see how they can also profitably help "de-market" obesity.[15]

1. **Think Extra-Small and Extra-Large.** Why do food companies supersize? From 1970 to 2000, the number of new larger-sized packages increased tenfold.[16] There are two reasons: 1) to satisfy our demand for value, and 2) to match the competition. There will always be people who want to be able to buy a lot of food for very little money. If only one restaurant provided supersized value meals, it would catch both our attention and our $3.59. If the competitor across the street didn't quickly do the same, they'd have to start closing up shop.[17]

   But while some of us want supersized values, others want smaller packages. We call these the "Portion Prone Segment." For instance, we found that half of the loyal users of one popular snack food said they would pay 15 percent more for a new package that helped them better control how much they ate. Although smaller packages would be more expensive (per ounce) compared to larger ones, this Portion Prone Segment would be willing to pay more to eat less . . . or to eat better. Given the $43 billion spent on diet foods and weight-loss programs each year, this is probably a big segment of people.

   Should companies abandon the value-priced supersize packages in favor of little boutique-size portion packs? Absolutely not. There are sizable markets for both—one that wants value and one that wants portion control. Some snack-food companies have started to capitalize on this with new 100-calorie packages.

2. **Create Packages with Pause Points.** Remember when we moved the candy dish six feet away from the secretaries and they ate half as many? They told us the six-foot distance gave them time to "pause" and ask themselves

whether they were really hungry. In the same way, building "pause points" into packaging can give people a chance to ask themselves if they really want to keep eating.

Pause points can be created by separating a large container into several smaller containers. For example, internal sleeves force us to actively make a decision to eat more. In the Lab, we call this "Thin Mint" packaging, in honor of the favorite Girl Scouts cookies. Instead of greeting us with a wide-open, no-serving-size-limit tray, Thin Mints are carefully wrapped in two cellophane sleeves. As much as you might want to overeat, when you hit the bottom of that first sleeve, it gives you pause. That's about all most of us need to stop. One of the more extreme versions of this principle can be found in Japan, where many brands sell individually packaged cookies.

Stopping points can take other forms. We showed this in one of our Lab's Red Chip studies. We took cans of Pringles (potato chips in a tube) and dyed every seventh chip red; in other cans, we dyed every fourteenth chip red; a last group of cans was left plain—no red chips. We then set up a video and invited people in to enjoy some Pringles. Those who ate from the cans where every seventh chip was red ate an average of 10. Those who ate from the cans where every fourteenth chip was red ate an average of 15 chips. Those with no red chips ate 23. Having something, almost anything, to interrupt our eating gives us the chance to decide if we want to continue.

Large multi-packs containing smaller individual servings also provide natural break points. We tested this concept when we gave 124 students either a large Ziploc bag containing 200 M&M's or a large Ziploc bag that, in turn, contained 10 smaller bags, each containing 20 M&M's. When there was only one bag to open, people ate an average of 73 M&M's during an hour. Those with the smaller bag usually ate a multiple of 10. When the hour was over, they had eaten an average of 42 each. Not a big deal? That's 112 calories less—the mindless margin.

3. **Change the Recipe, but Keep It Good.** Since the whimpering phaseout of McDonald's McLean sandwich in 1996, food marketers across the United States and beyond have taken the wrong lesson away from McLean's McFailure. It wasn't that there was no market for healthy foods or that companies just can't make good low-fat products. What needs to be realized is that these foods were typically new products that tasted *new,* were advertised as *new,* and were expected (by us) to sacrifice taste to virtue. In contrast to this "Look at this!" approach, companies could quietly alter existing products in modest ways that reduce caloric density. This would bypass negative expectations and give healthier products a fair shot.

These silent, healthy changes are something my Lab calls "stealth health."

Just as Mikey in the Life cereal ads didn't want to eat anything that was good for him, we too have our suspicions of any food that is supposed to healthy. With stealth health, small formulation changes can gradually trim away the calories without our ever even knowing it happened. We taste pretty much what we expect to taste— the same, good-ole-tasting candy bar or frozen dinner.

In general, we use the size of a food as an indicator of "value." That is, the bigger the food, the better the value.

The Conspiracy That Isn't

A few times each year a journalist calls me hoping to write a story on food-industry conspiracies. When I ask for the specific examples that are motivating their story, most "examples" have less nefarious explanations. Do supermarkets put the meat department in the back so we make more impulse purchases en route? The more practical explanation: That's where the power supply, the plumbing, and the loading docks are located, and nobody wants to see those in the *front* of the store.

Someone recently asked, "If a single Pop-Tart is one serving, why do Pop-Tarts come two to a package?" They presupposed that once the package is opened, Kellogg's wants us to eat both of them. Ergo, Kellogg's wants us all to be fat—Pop-Tart packages are proof of this!

Now let's hear from Bill Post, the plant manager who produced the first Pop-Tart:

> The packaging equipment was expensive. To package them singly would have required twice as many machines. Kellogg's didn't want to invest in a lot of machines until they knew how it would sell.[18]

Practical, cost-based explanations motivate many food-marketing decisions. This is unfortunate for Upton Sinclair wannabes. A cost-based explanation is never as interesting as a good conspiracy story.

While adding water, or air, or filler may do little to the taste of the candy bar or frozen dinner, it helps maintain the perception of value, and it decreases calorie levels. Even if such efforts only reduce calorie levels by 10 percent, a 10 percent decrease in our daily calorie consumption would either slow or reverse the weight gain among most of us. It's important to remember, however, that this would be a slow process. It would be a pound-by-pound loss, just as it was a pound-by-pound gain.

Here are three facts about slightly modified and reformulated foods: 1) When the calorie density of a food is decreased, we eat the same volume we usually do, 2) we think we are just as full, and 3) we think the food tastes just as good (as long as it hasn't been labeled "reduced calorie" or "healthy").

4. **Provide Simple Labels, but Don't Be Too Optimistic.** "Education." It is the one-word easy-out answer to anything related to health. Once we say we need more "education," it becomes somebody else's problem—like government's or industry's. And if their education efforts don't work? The answer is, "Do more."

Marketing nutrition is a noble enterprise, but as I researched a professional book on this topic (*Marketing Nutrition*), it became very clear to me that education—as defined by most experts—was *not* the answer. We are either too busy or too distracted to read packages, or we are too preoccupied or hungry to care that we should eat a carrot stick rather than a handful of Doritos.

Clearly labeling calories and serving sizes is a good idea. But we need to be realistic about how much impact it will have on behavior. Most research shows that—outside of an artificial lab situation—labeling influences only a small minority of consumers. Still, it's worth having.

The question is, where should this information stop? In my work with an FDA-sponsored committee in 2005–

2006, a major recommendation on the issue of away-from-home labeling of food was that companies emphasize calories. That is the one common denominator most widely understood.

If the answer isn't nutrition education, what is it? That is where mindfully reengineering our personal environment comes in. Once that is done, the burden of knowing and doing changes dramatically.

5. **Keep It Affordable.** Generally, when prices go up, consumption goes down. This is true with meat and fresh produce, but it doesn't seem to be true with those indulging "C" foods—candy, cookies, cake, and ice cream. Within a reasonable range, when the price of these items goes up, we either buy them anyway or switch to another brand.[19] Some studies have shown that increasing the price of selected vending-machine candy caused people to buy less of that candy. This works primarily in limited-choice environments such as schools, however. In most situations, if the price of a candy bar went up by 25¢, people would either pay it or they would buy a different brand. They wouldn't stop eating candy. Similarly, if a fast-food restaurant raised its prices, people wouldn't stop eating fast food, they would simply eat it somewhere else. Raising prices doesn't make people eat healthier, it makes them go to a competitor and eat the same food. A "sin tax" isn't a "stopping tax," it's a "shopping tax."

What is certain is that large increases in food prices make us shop for alternatives. It doesn't mean that we look for healthier options, it doesn't change our food desires, it just changes where we would go to buy our french fries and candy bars. Raising prices within a reasonable free-market range doesn't change behavior, it penalizes the people with the least money.

Our challenge is to make the healthier options more attractive and more affordable. We cannot legislate or tax people into eating brussels sprouts. That is not to say that a smart, well-intentioned marketer can't convince them.

21st-Century Marketing

The 19th century has been called the Century of Hygiene. More lives were saved or extended due to an improved understanding of hygiene and public health than by any other single cause. We learned that rats were not house pets and that it's a good idea for doctors to wash their hands before surgery.

The 20th century was the Century of Medicine. Vaccines, antibiotics, transfusions, and chemotherapy all helped contribute to longer, healthier lives. In 1900, the life expectancy of an American was 49 years. In 2000, it was 77 years.

I believe the 21st century will be the Century of Behavior Change. Medicine is still making fundamental discoveries that can fight disease, but changing everyday, long-term behavior is the key to adding years and quality to our lives. This will involve reducing risky behavior and making changes in exercise and nutrition. There isn't a simple prescription that can be written for such behavior change. Eating better and exercising more are decisions we need to be motivated to make.

When it comes to contributing to the life span and quality of life in the next couple of generations, smart marketers could pick up the banner and lead the charge. Using creativity, they can develop healthy foods that are more enjoyable to eat and products that make it less onerous to exercise. Using persuasion, they can encourage us to get off the couch, eat better, and move more.

In the end, nobody can motivate us to change but ourselves. But a well-intentioned marketer can make the job easier for us to start.

Reengineering Strategy #9: Portion-Size Me

The McSubway study gave us a number of ideas we can take to the drive-through.

- **Beware of the health halo.** The better the food, the worse the extras. People eating "low-fat" granola ate 21 percent more calories, and those eating "healthy" at Subway rewarded themselves by ordering cheese, mayo, chips, and cookies. Who really overeats—the guy who knows he's eating 710 calories at McDonald's, or the woman who thinks she's eating a 350-calorie Subway meal that actually contains 500 calories?
- **Think small or super-share.** Supersizing may seem like a bargain, but most refills are free anyway, and a large bag of fries will be cold by the time you get to the greasy bottom. Is the medium size still too large for you? Take some fries and toss

them out on your way to the table. You'll get the taste you want without overdoing it. But here's the real value—split a value meal combo and order an extra drink. Half a sandwich and half the fries. But hold the cookie.

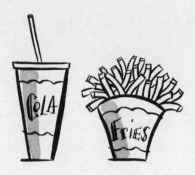

10

Mindlessly Eating Better

WHEN WE'RE FREEWHEELING DOWN an 80-foot-long cereal aisle, or deciding which of 16 pizza toppings we want, or asking to see the cheesecake menu, it's easy to forget world history. In 75 years Americans have gone from huddling in Depression breadlines to hoarding food-ration stamps to helping feed a starving, war-torn, pre-McDonald's Europe.[1]

Today the food table has turned.

High at the 30,000-foot level, critics blame low prices and easily available food for helping make us fat.[2] Some blame government subsidies to agriculture, supersizing food companies, and even the schools. Others blame the inactivity encouraged by cars, elevators, computers, garage-door openers, and PlayStations.[3] If all of these were gone, our environment clearly would be less "obesigenic." Would we all revert to having the sleek, trim figures of people we see in 1950s black-and-white photos? That is less clear. Changing capitalism and changing the world are slow processes. And when it comes to food, it's not clear how much of the world wants to change.

At the other extreme, at ground level, the emphasis is on individual responsibility and bite-by-bite diligence. Here we see people counting calories, carbs, and fat grams and moving nomadically from diet to diet. It's hard not to feel the frustration of friends and family when their love of life is weighed down by having to estimate the calories in the salad dressing they have "on the side," or in the baloney-thin slice of birthday cake they carefully cut. With more than 200 daily decisions to make about food, this much micro-thinking can joylessly grind a person down.

Neither of these extremes holds bright promise for the person who wants to get her family or herself back on the right track (and maybe back into some of her "signal clothes"). One approach is slow, difficult, and unlikely to work; the other is all-consuming and prone to relapse.

All my research suggests that the key to change lies in the middle.[4] We may not be able to outlaw every drive-through restaurant or tax every pint of ice cream in our community, but we can reengineer our personal food environment to help us and our families eat better.[5] We can turn the food in our life from being a temptation or a regret to something we guiltlessly enjoy. We can move from mindless overeating to mindless *better* eating.

The Modest Goal of Better Eating

Better eating means different things to different people. It can mean eating less, eating without guilt, eating more nutritiously, or eating with greater enjoyment. This is the *good* type of mindless eating.

Eating Better Is Best

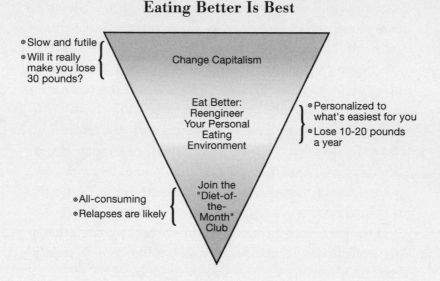

Each year when I pay my annual dues to the American Dietetic Association, I log on to their website: www.Eat Right.org.[6] It's a great website, and eating right is a great goal. The problem is that it's just too daunting for most of us. It seems so absolute and so joyless. But the idea of eating *better* is do-able. While eating *right* is a long-term goal, eating *better* is something we can start today. Eating better entails small steps. It leads us back to the mindless margin of Chapter 1.

Our body and our mind fight against deprivation diets that cut our daily calorie intake from 2,000 to 1,200 calories a day. But they don't really notice a 100–200 calorie difference because they're not as sensitive within this range—it doesn't ring the starvation alarm in our body's metabolism.

We can trim these calories out of our day relatively easily. The key is to do it unknowingly. To *mindlessly* eat better. To reach this goal, we need to reengineer our mindless margin.

Reengineering Your Mindless Margin

In early 2006, I gave a research presentation at a prestigious medical school. Afterward, an epidemiologist asked, "I now see what causes people to mindlessly overeat, but what are the top three tips I can give my patients so they can eat less?"

The quest to find the "Top Three Secret Tips" of weight loss is what sells thousands of magazines in the supermarket checkout line every day. Yet this quest is frustrating because there aren't any one-size-fits-all answers.

Each chapter in *Mindless Eating* has suggested small adjustments you can make to your eating environment—ways you can reengineer it to avoid being trapped by an extra 100 calories here or there. This allows you to choose changes that are specifically relevant and motivating for you. For instance, one fast-food-loving colleague who tended to mindlessly overeat at lunch reengineered his mindless margin with three food trade-offs: 1) "No potato chips unless I've exercised that day," 2) "Throw half my French fries away before I sit down," 3) "I can eat a dessert only if I go back and buy it *after* I've finished eating my whole lunch."

Reengineering Your Food Environment

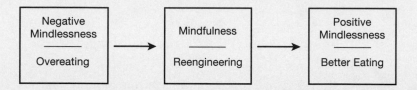

There is no tip sheet in the world that would have specified these three personalized positive changes. This is the power of knowing the basic principles in this book and adapting them to fit your specific situation.[7]

Here are two more techniques for putting these principles to work: food trade-offs and food policies.

Food Trade-Offs Food trade-offs state, "I can eat x if I do y." For example, I can eat dessert if I've worked out; I can have chips if I don't have a morning snack; I can have movie popcorn if I have only a salad for dinner; I can have a second soft drink if I use the stairs all day.

Food trade-offs are great because we don't have to deny ourselves a food we love. We just have to make a small concession in the name of good health. Food trade-offs also put us back in charge of our food decisions by raising the "price we pay" for overeating.

Look at my lunchtime colleague—all three of his tips are related to food trade-offs. If he wanted potato chips, he had to exercise (a trade-off). If he wanted more French fries, he'd either have to buy more or borrow some from a dining mate (a very tacky trade-off). If he wanted a dessert after lunch, he had to get up and buy it (a pause point trade-off).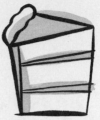

Food Policies The low-carb diet was initially successful because people didn't have to make repeated decisions in the face of temptation. Many summarized the diet in one sentence: "Eat meat and vegetables, but nothing else." This was a food policy. No need for "just this once" decision making, it was a personal rule. No exceptions.

Food policies are great because you can personalize them to your situation. They come in many different forms: serve myself 20 percent less than I usually would; no second helpings of any starch; never eat at my desk; only eat snacks that don't come in wrappers; no bagels on weekdays; only half-size desserts. Food policies don't involve any trade-offs, they just eliminate one or two habits that have mindlessly encroached on our lifestyle. We don't have to commit to big sacrifices, we only have to pick the habits we can easily forgo.

The Power of Three

What three 100-calorie changes in your daily food routine would be easiest for you to turn into mindlessly *positive* eating habits?[8]

Why only three? As I have said, most diets fail because

Your Mindful Eating Plan
Key Points

- **Your Mindless Margin.** By making 100–200 calorie changes in your daily intake, you won't feel deprived and backslide.
- **Mindless Better Eating.** Focus on reengineering small behaviors that will move you from mindless overeating to mindless better eating. Five common places to look (diet danger zones) include meals, snacks, parties, restaurants, and your desk or dashboard.
- **Mindful Reengineering.** To trim your mindless margin, you can use basic diet tips, but a more personalized approach is to use 1) food trade-offs, or 2) food policies. Both give you a chance to eat some of what you want without making it a belabored decision.
- **The Power of Three.** Design three easy, do-able changes that you can mindlessly make without much sacrifice.
- **Mindless Margin Checklist.** Use this daily checklist to help you move from mindless overeating to mindless better eating.

they ask us to do too much. Three small changes is reasonable. If we make three small, 100-calorie changes, by the end of the year we'll be as much as 30 pounds lighter than if we didn't make them. Even if you only succeed in making one or two of them, you are still going to weigh 10 to 20 pounds less in a year. If you try for three a day, and you hit two, you still have reason to smile and hold your head high.

Experts in behavioral modification say it takes about 28 days—one month—to break an old habit and replace it with a good one. That is, if you can stop biting your finger-nails for 28 consecutive days, the next 28 days will be much, much easier, because you will be over the hump. I suppose you might still get fingernail cravings, but the patterns and the associations that led you to bite them off in the past will have been changed. The same is true with food.

That leaves just one problem: How do you remind your-self to make these three changes for 28 days running? You could simply say, "Oh, I'll remember," but it's too easy to slip.[9] We need to be held accountable, otherwise we fall back into our normal patterns.

This is where the Power of Three checklist comes in. This is simply a piece of paper that has a month's worth of days across the top (1–31) and your three daily 100-calorie changes written down the side. Every evening, you check off the changes you've accomplished. This small act of account-ability makes you more mindful throughout the day. And every check mark is its own small reward. Not every day will be perfect, but the idea is to slowly start building the right habits. If these are 100-calorie changes, 32 checks each month should equal about a pound of weight. And if you can make 28 consistent checks for one new behavior, you are well on your way to establishing a *positive* mindless eating habit.

Imagine a friend whose major dietary trap is meal stuff-ing.[10] If we look at this person's Power of Three checklist be-low, we see that over the course of the month, her record was not perfect. On some days, like the fourth, she didn't make any changes, and on the eighth day she only made one. Yet over the course of the month, there were 27 days on which she used the Half-Plate Rule; there were 13 days when she started last and finished last; and there were 24 days when she only served vegetables family-style (and left the rest of the food on the stove). If she had eaten as usual, and if each item added 100 calories to her monthly chow time, she would have eaten 6,400 calories extra [(27+13+24) x 100], which is about a two-pound difference. While it wasn't a perfect month, she should be pleased. Making positive changes that become mindless is the goal.

The Power of Three Checklist

MARCH	1	2	3	4	5	6	7	8	9	10	11	...	31	TOTAL
Use the Half-Plate rule - half veggies or salad	x	x	x		x	x	x	x	x		x		x	27
Slow down - start last, finish last		x			x			x	x				x	13
Only serve vegetables "family style"	x	x	x		x	x	x		x	x	x		x	24

If she also had a secondary weakness with desktop dining, she could have replaced one of her three checklist items with a snack-related change, such as "Drink no more than one sugared soft drink." But it's important to limit yourself initially to three changes. Three changes are manageable.

The more you can focus, the more you can feel a small sense of victory when you have a perfect day. You can always make more changes after these habits have become mindless.

It's easy, positive, and slow. It's empowering. It's choosing what you want to do and what you think you can do well.

The Tyranny of the Moment

We can commit to making a small change in life, such as not eating sweet snacks before dinner. We can write it down, cross our heart, and announce it to others. We can really, really mean it. But fast-forward two days. It was a hectic day at work, you finished a 45-minute commute, you're drained, and you know a frozen Snickers bar is waiting in the left-hand corner of the freezer door. It's easy to break your cross-the-heart commitment. After all, today is an exception—it was a tough day, and come to think of it, you didn't have a very big breakfast. Your Mindful Eating Plan has just been thwarted by the tyranny of the moment. And the moment—this one exceptional moment—tyrannically wins every time.

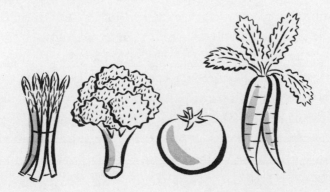

Sometimes that inner voice says, "I know I said I'm not going to eat out of vending machines at work, but today's different—it's been crazy," or "I know I still have to do my sit-ups today, but it's late—I'll do twice as many tomorrow when I wake up," or "I know I should've had only one glass of wine, but this is a really great dinner and a really great wine."

There's only one thing that's strong enough to defeat the tyranny of the moment.

Habit.

As mentally disciplined as most of us like to think we are, nothing beats having to face facts each night and check off a little box. We have very selective memories, but the Power of Three Checklist lets us know just why—or why not—we have painlessly lost two pounds on the thirty-first of the month.

The First Step Toward Home

Suppose you found yourself two miles from home without a ride. Although you could get home three times faster if you ran, most people would settle for walking. Running wouldn't be worth the sweat and discomfort, and walking will get you there at a reasonable and painless rate. Each step brings you a little closer, and before you know it, you are halfway home and still moving forward.

It's the same with mindlessly losing weight. It need not be a sweaty, painful sprint.[11] It can be a slow, steady walk that begins with removing unwanted eating cues and rearranging your home, office, and eating habits so they work for you and your family rather than against you. These comfortable steps will add up—one or two pounds a month. Before long you'll find yourself at home.

The best diet is the one you don't know you're on.

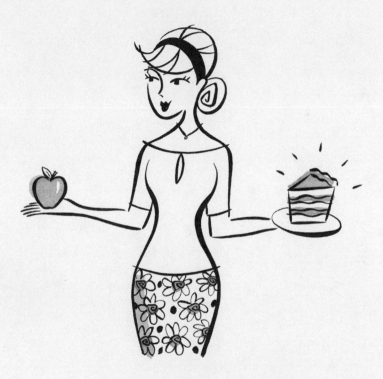

Appendix A

Comparing Popular Diets

DESCRIPTION	ADVANTAGES	DISADVANTAGES

SOUTH BEACH DIET
Developed by Arthur Agatston, M.D., to help patients with heart and cardiovascular problems.

•The theory: You can still eat fats and carbs—but the *right* fats and the *right* carbs. •Involves radically cutting down on fat and carbs, except those found in whole grains, fruits, and vegetables. •Works in three phases. Phase one is a strict two-week period prohibiting many foods, which may lead to rapid weight loss of up to 13 pounds. The second phase reintroduces some restricted foods as weight loss slows down to goal weight. The third phase is a maintenance level that reintroduces moderate amounts of formerly restricted foods.	•Nutritionally balanced after the initial phase. •Does not rely on high levels of saturated fat. •No calorie or fat counting. •Encourages regular meals and snacks. •Provides simple recipes.	•Very demanding for those accustomed to carb-rich diets. •Can be expensive and time-consuming. •Must be a new way of life. Many find it constricting. •Carb restriction may be difficult for dieters who exercise vigorously.

DESCRIPTION	ADVANTAGES	DISADVANTAGES

SUGAR BUSTERS DIET
Developed by a group of M.D.'s and the CEO of a Fortune 500 energy company.

•The theory: Sugar is toxic to our bodies. It causes an increase in insulin, which causes weight gain. •Recommends a daily calorie intake split into a 40/30/30: 40 percent fat, 30 percent protein, and 30 percent carbohydrates. •Prohibits refined sugar and starches that rank high in the Glycemic Index (GI), such as potatoes and pasta.	•Helps to eliminate consumption of refined sugar. •Does not involve calorie counting. •Eliminates many foods that are clearly unhealthy. •Encourages exercise.	•Eliminates some valuable minerals and nutrients. •Not suitable for vegetarians. •Weight loss is probably due to the automatic calorie reduction and not the 40/30/30 ratio.

WEIGHT WATCHERS POINTS DIET
Developed by Weight Watchers International.

•The theory: As long as you stay within your point limit, you can eat whatever you want. •Assigns a point value to all foods. •Dieters are weighed on a weekly basis and then advised on how many daily points they should aim to consume for the coming week.	•Does not exclude major food groups. •Suitable for vegetarians. •Teaches portion control and nutrition. •Makes it easy to dine out. •Support is offered in the form of weekly meetings.	•Membership can become expensive over time. •Weight loss may be slower than with other diets. •Points can be "spent" on unhealthy foods. •Must know exact serving size to calculate point value.

DESCRIPTION	ADVANTAGES	DISADVANTAGES
THE ZONE DIET Developed by Barry Sears, M.D.		
•The theory: Managing your insulin levels through diet can lead to weight loss. •Recommends daily calorie intake be split into a 40/30/30 ratio: 40 percent carbohydrates, 30 percent protein, 30 percent fat. •Sticking to the precalculated ratios will help control insulin levels, which in turn will speed up the fat-burning process. •The amount of food eaten is also an important factor in this diet, and dieters are encouraged to carefully assess and monitor their food portions.	•Teaches good eating habits such as portion control and sugar reduction. •Allows for a fruit-and-vegetable-rich diet. •Allows some carbohydrate intake, and cravings begin to disappear after a few days. •Can yield rapid weight loss for special occasions, like weddings or reunions.	•Rapid weight loss is often swiftly followed by weight gain. •Not practical for many people and some report it is difficult to fit around lifestyle. •Can be expensive to follow. •Restrictions involve cutting out some valuable vitamins and minerals. •Time-consuming.
ATKINS DIET Developed by Robert C. Atkins, M.D.		
•The theory: Weight gain isn't caused by fat or portion size—it's caused by the way our bodies deal with the breakdown of processed and starchy carbohydrates. •Very high protein allows virtually no carbohydrates, particularly during the initial stages. •By cutting out carbohydrates, dieters will go into a state where their bodies begin to burn off stored fat. •After the initial stage, the diet provides a maintenance program, which gradually reintroduces limited carbohydrates into the diet.	•Promotes rapid weight loss. •Enables dieters to eat unlimited protein-rich and high-fat foods. •Has been proven effective. •Quick and inexpensive.	•Very restrictive. •Condones high consumption of saturated fats. •Can cause bad breath, nausea, and headaches, particularly in the initial stage. •Cuts out many valuable nutrients. •Not suitable for vegetarians. •Raises concerns about long-term effects of such high levels of protein and fat upon vital organs.

DESCRIPTION	ADVANTAGES	DISADVANTAGES
YOUR MINDFUL EATING PLAN		
•The theory: Making 100 to 200 calorie changes in our daily food intake can lead to weight loss of up to 10 to 20 pounds over the course of a year.	•Easy and inexpensive.	•Weight loss is gradual.
•Focuses on reengineering the hidden persuaders that cause us to eat more than we think we ate or want to eat.	•No hunger or deprivation.	•Until small changes become second nature, this works best when a daily habit checklist is used.
•Trim your mindless margin by using 1) food trade-offs, or 2) food policies. Both give you the chance to eat some of what you want.	•Easy to use with family members.	•Personalizing the plan requires introspection and thought.
•The Power of Three: Design three easy, do-able changes that you can mindlessly make without much sacrifice.	•No foods are off-limits, but portions are reduced.	
•After determining key diet danger areas, a personalized daily habit checklist is designed to help you mindlessly lose 100 to 300 calories a day.	•Can fit any routine; flexible to what a person thinks will be easiest for him or her.	
	•Can be combined with diets.	
	•Weight stays off.	

Appendix B

Defusing Your Diet Danger Zones

The Diet Danger Zones are traps that catch all of us at one time or another, but most people fall into only one or two on a regular basis. Do you see yourself in the descriptions below?

#1. The Meal Stuffer
Stuffers eat primarily during mealtimes, but then they eat to excess, cleaning everything on their plate. They often eat so quickly that they're uncomfortably full after they finish. Meal stuffers consider themselves to have "healthy appetites." They often take second helpings at home.

#2. The Snack Grazer
Grazers reach for whatever food is available, typically about three times a day. While they love the 4 C's, convenience is usually more important to them than taste. They seldom pass up a candy dish. For these people, snacking can be a nervous habit, something that gives

them an excuse to get up and walk around, or something they can do with their hands while watching TV or reading. They might be hungry when they snack, but it's almost done more out of habit than hunger.

#3. The Party Binger
Parties—buffets, receptions, tailgates, and happy hours—these are high-distraction environments where the food is the backdrop for either business or fun, and it's easy to lose track of how much they've eaten or drunk. Party bingers are often professionals who frequently wine and dine, or single, stay-out-late young people.

#4. The Restaurant Indulger
While many of us eat lunch away from home, the restaurant indulger also eats dinner out at least three days a week. Like party bingers, restaurant indulgers are often on an expense account. They may also be affluent gourmets or DINKs (double income, no kids) in their thirty-something years.

#5. The Desktop Diner (or Dashboard Diner)
Both speed-eat while multi-tasking at their desk or in their car. Desktop diners eat at their desk partly to save time, but more often to save the hassle of getting a real lunch. It's not that they're overly busy—they're under-motivated. If the right person were to stop by to ask them to lunch, they'd probably go. But more often, they snack out of the vending machine or grab a donut from the mail room.

Now that you've identified your diet danger zones, what can you do? Let's look at five composites of people and some of the mindless eating changes they could make to defuse their diet danger zones.

1. **For Meal Stuffers . . . Design a Different Dinner.** Ever since he and his wife married 22 years ago, Peter has pretty much been the cook of the house. He loves making food, he loves gardening, and he loves to eat dinner . . . a little too much. Although his wife has been able to stay trim over the years, Peter and his two teenage daughters have both found that their weight has steadily grown. For a while, Peter attributed his increasing weight to turning 50 and to his "slowing metabolism," and he justified the weight gain of his girls as "growth spurts." But even though all three of them are above average height, they're getting bulky.

   The notion of a diet or even watching what he ate seemed a bit too feminine to Peter, and he didn't want to sacrifice much to get things back on track. A halfhearted attempt at an exercise program lasted about five days. If something was going to work for him, it needed to be easy and convenient. It couldn't be seen as a diet. The dinner needed to be tasty—not steamed vegetables and four ounces of boiled fish.

   Peter didn't want to make his daughters self-conscious about their weight and about dieting. He loves that his wife never talks about her weight.

   The meal stuffer needs to design a different dinner. Meal stuffing is a common problem with men, and it's worse at the evening meal. Choosing three of the following changes is something Peter could easily do. After the

first month, he wouldn't even notice the difference—
except in his weight.

- Preplate the high-calorie foods in the kitchen and
  leave the leftovers there. Do not serve what some
  call "fat-family" style, unless it's veggies and salad.
- Keep dinner classy by using nice dishes, but use
  smaller plates and taller glasses.
- Manage the pace. Slow down, so appetites can catch
  up with what's been eaten. Slow music can help.
- Avoid having too many foods on the table. The
  more variety there is, the more people will eat.
- Get into the habit of leaving something on the
  plate.
- Eat fruit for dessert instead of more indulgent
  choices.
- Adopt the Half-Plate Rule. Half the plate is filled
  with vegetables and the other half is protein and
  starch.

2. **For Snack Grazers . . . Avoid Snack Traps.** Tracy
   prides herself on being a reasonably healthy cook. Her
   husband's family has a history of heart problems and Tracy
   has adjusted her cooking habits to accommodate his diet,
   and everyone has benefited. When Tracy had their second
   son, she thought she might take a break from work and
   stay with the boys until they started school.

   Although Tracy has a big frame, her weight was pretty
   much under control until she decided to quit work. At
   that point, she was home most of the day and preparing
   food more often than before. Although the meals were

still balanced and well portioned, she was trapped between meals by snacks—the candy dish, the half-eaten
pint of chocolate ice cream in the freezer, the cookies that
call for her when she gets too close to the cupboard.

It's important for Tracy to remember that we often
snack not because we're hungry, but because it's part of a
script ("I'll turn on the TV and then look for something to
eat"). If we keep snacks out of the TV room and out of the
computer room, we'll be able to better interrupt those
scripts.

There are a number of other changes Tracy could consider to avoid snack traps. Any combination of them
could keep her eating within her mindless margin of
trimming down 100–200 calories a day.

- Think "Back." For all those foods that aren't good
  for you, think "Back." Put them in the back of the
  cupboard, in the back of the refrigerator, or in the
  back of the freezer. Keep these tempting goodies
  wrapped in aluminum foil.
- Do not "prebuy" snacks for a future occasion. If
  you must buy snacks, buy those your family likes
  but you don't.
- If you get a craving, think of a substitute. Crunchy
  things like fruits and precut vegetables work for
  some people. Each week, buy a colorful variety of
  vegetables, precut them, and store them on the first
  or second shelf of the refrigerator.
- Chewing gum can distract you away from the 4 C's:
  chips, cookies, ice cream, and candy.
- Only eat at the table—the one in the kitchen or the

one in the dining room. Don't wolf things down over the sink or in front of an open refrigerator.

- Keep the tempting foods out of sight and out of mind. Store them in the basement, or in the back of out-of-the-way cupboards. Repack mini-portions of them into Ziploc bags or Tupperware so you can't see them and they can't tempt you like those Hershey's Kisses in the clear glass jars.
- If family members want different foods, have separate cupboards that are assigned to them and off-limits to you.
- The only food that should be out on the counter are the healthy foods. Substitute a fruit dish for your cookie jar.
- Never eat directly from a package. Always portion food out into a dish so you must face exactly how much you'll eat.

3. **For Party Bingers . . . Party Less Hearty.** Within a span of 10 years, David had been given three promotions and had made two big moves, to be nearly at the top of his profession while still in his 50s. That was the good news. The bad news was that his position required him to entertain and to be entertained at receptions, parties, and buffets four to five nights a week. Within two years, the combined stress of the new job and the almost daily receptions had made him look like a different—and much bigger—man.

Part of the reward for spending so much time working was the eating. There was a lot of good food, and he compensated for being away from home by eating a little more than he should. But "a little more" four or five days a week added up to exactly 23 pounds in three years.

The small changes he chooses can take this weight back. Not by next Tuesday, but very possibly within a year. None of these changes will "put David out" or make him feel deprived. They might make him a little more focused on people, on business, or even on having fun.

- Stay more than an arm's length away from the buffet tables and snack bowls.
- Put only two items on your plate during any given trip to the table.
- Use the volume approach to make yourself feel full. Chow down on the big healthy stuff (like broccoli and carrots) and then see if you have room for the rest.
- When you think you'll be distracted by an important (or fun) conversation, set the food down and give the conversation your full attention. Remember, the more you focus on people (and distractions like the Super Bowl on TV), the more you'll tend to eat.
- As you enter the room, tell yourself you're there first to conduct business and secondarily to eat. Be aware that tension or nervousness may be prompting you to refill your plate or your glass. The fact that this is not comfort food—you're there for business, not pleasure—may strengthen your resolve to eat less or lighter food.
- If you plan to attend a cocktail party or a buffet-

style dinner, arrive late or leave early. If you arrive late, most of the good stuff will be gone by the time you show up. Leave early and you'll make it easier to avoid a second (or third) helping of dessert.

4. **For Restaurant Indulgers . . . Develop Restaurant Rules.** Carmen's cosmopolitan. She's a fun, single, energetic 28-year-old lover of life. She has a job she enjoys, "enough" money, and lots of friends she likes to keep up with. A basic day for Carmen entails skipping breakfast, meeting a friend for lunch, working until 7:00 or so, and then meeting other friends or a date for dinner. She hardly ever cooks for herself (only for dinner parties), but her life is filled with great food because she eats out nearly every meal.

Carmen used to like to think of herself as voluptuous and secretly prided herself on looking like a "real woman." Over the past four years, however, her weight has become more and more of an issue. She finds herself wearing looser clothes and passing on the rewarding types of clothes that used to get her "second looks" a few years back.

The restaurant indulger needs to develop restaurant rules. The following changes would be enough to help Carmen take off 10 or more pounds in a year. Although it might also work for the rest of us, we don't get these big results if we don't eat out very often.

- Use the Rule of Two: Limit yourself to two of the following: an appetizer, a drink, or a dessert. Pick any two.
- If the bread basket is on the table, you are going to

eat bread. Either ask the waiter to forget it or to take it away early. You can also keep passing it so it stays on the other side of the table.

• Before you start to eat, ask the waiter to prewrap half of your entrée to take home. That way you will not be tempted to polish it off as soon as it arrives.

• Ask for water and alternate glasses of water with glasses of whatever else you're drinking.

• Sit next to the person you think will be the slowest eater at the table. Use him or her as a pacesetter. Always be the last one to start eating, and set your fork down after every bite.

• If you want dessert, see if someone will share it. The best part of a dessert is the first two bites.

5. **For Desktop and Dashboard Diners . . . Change Gears.** Paul works in a cubicle-filled office building that he refers to as "Dilbert, Inc." He's 47, but at home he feels 27 and at work he feels 67. He adores his wife and teenage daughter, but he isn't especially crazy about his job or colleagues. He usually sleeps in and delays going into work until the last second, grabs coffee and a bagel at a convenience store during his drive, and works through lunch rather than trying to rustle up a lunch mate and risking a lot of boring shoptalk. (Besides, he thinks it makes him look dedicated.)

The upshot is that Paul snacks all day long from "vending machine alley," on mailroom and lunchroom leftovers, and on the PowerBars and M&M's he keeps in his desk. By the time he gets home to his family, he is ready to unwind over a big dinner. After all, he hasn't had a "real meal" yet today—only 1,500 calories consumed on the run. No wonder his work clothes are feeling increasingly uncomfortable.

Desktop and dashboard diners can choose the changes below that seem like the easiest and most practical to make:

- Brown-bag it. Even if you only do this a couple of times a week, you're ahead of the game because you're in more control of your food choices.
- Stock your desk or lunchroom refrigerator with yogurt and pop-top cans of tuna fish. Protein can take the edge off a snack attack.
- Turn off the computer or pull the car over while you eat. If you focus on what you're eating, you might even discover that you don't really like vending-machine or convenience-store food.
- Use food policies and food trade-offs. For example: the first thing you eat at work is fruit; eating an indulgent snack means taking a walk during your break.
- Chew gum to prevent eating from boredom or stress.
- Replace every other soft drink with water. Offices tend to be dry. We often think we're hungry when instead we're simply thirsty. Fill up your water bottle a number of times each day.

Notes

Introduction: The Science of Snacking

1. The average person initially believes they only make about 15 food-related decisions per day. See Brian Wansink and Jeffrey Sobal, "Hidden Persuaders and 200 Daily Decisions," *Environment and Behavior* (2007), forthcoming; and Brian Wansink and Collin R. Payne, "Daily Food Decisions and Estimation Biases" (2006), under review at *Psychological Reports.*

2. See "Out of the Frying Pan, Into the Fryer," *The Economist* 330:7486 (Jan. 15, 1994) 89, which reported how government research scientists are sometimes hired out for civilian business use.

3. The labs mentioned here are only a few of the many, but they're the ones that influenced my thinking the most. Some labs, like those run by C. Peter Herman, Janet Polivy, and Patty Pliner at the University of Toronto have generated many foundational insights over the past 35 years. The labs of Carol Bisogni, David Levitsky, Jeffrey Sobal, Carol Devine, and Christine Olson at Cornell have challenged conventional thinking related to issues of family dining, college weight gain, and the impact of breakfast on how much we eat. Other labs, such as Kelly Brownell's at Yale, have produced the insights related to

clinical treatment of the obese. Paul Rozin's lab at the University of Pennsylvania has given us most of our insights about food fears and neophobia. James O. Hill's Center at the University of Colorado is examining how food and exercise relate, and Dennis Bier's lab at the Baylor Medical School focuses on the use of psychology to understand childhood obesity.

4. See Barbara Rolls and Robert Barnett, *The Volumetrics Weight-Control Plan* (New York: HarperTorch, 2000) and Barbara Rolls, *The Volumetrics Eating Plan: Techniques and Recipes for Feeling Full on Fewer Calories* (New York: HarperCollins, 2005).

5. See Herbert L. Meiselman and Howard G. Schutz, "History of Food Acceptance Research in the US Army," *Appetite* 40: 3 (June 2003): 199–216.

6. We have a pro-choice mission. It's "to conduct and disseminate quality research that *helps people use food to be who they want to be.*" For some people this could involve eating less, eating more nutritiously, or eating in a way that enables them to better enjoy their food. For health professionals and companies, this means designing ideas for changes that can help them more effectively help their clients or customers use food in a productive way. For administrators involved in food aid, this means giving them ideas that help their food-distribution efforts be more effective.

7. Until a few years ago, most research in business schools, and often research that related to sensory studies and food intake, was given a general class of approval or exemption. This was given as long as the research didn't threaten the participants, and as long as they gave their consent and could quit the study at any time. Because of litigation related to medical school research, such exemptions are no longer possible.

8. Some participants enjoy being part of a pool of people who are repeatedly involved in studies. We call this the "Food Psychology Panel," and its size has fluctuated between 300 and 3,000 over the past 20 years. Unlike most of the participants

in our studies, we don't eliminate these people's contact information. At their request, we keep them "in the loop" about new studies and by sending them newsletters as to what we are learning and how they can apply this in their lives.

1. The Mindless Margin

1. See Brian Wansink, "Environmental Factors that Increase the Food Intake and Consumption Volume of Unknowing Consumers," *Annual Review of Nutrition* 24 (2004): 455–79.
2. On average, those given the medium-size bucket ate 61.1 grams, while those given the large bucket ate 93.5 grams. Nobody finished all of their popcorn, which had been popped in partially hydrogenated (meaning "bad" trans fats) canola oil. This study was filmed for the ABC News' *Morning Edition*. It can be viewed at www.MindlessEating.org. See Brian Wansink and SeaBum Park, "At the Movies: How External Cues and Perceived Taste Impact Consumption Volume," *Food Quality and Preference,* 12:1(January 2001): 69–74.
3. The Spice Box can be found in Bevier Hall on the campus of the University of Illinois in Urbana. It's open January through April, and reservations can be made by calling 1-217-333-6520. It now serves dinner on Tuesdays and Fridays. The article described here is: Brian Wansink, Collin Payne, Jill North, and James E. Painter, "Fine as North Dakota Wine: Sensory Experiences and Food Intake," under review at *Physiology and Behavior*.
4. Special mega-cudos to Jill North, co-author and manager of the Fine Dining Program. After we designed the study, designed the labels, purchased the wine, and set up the experimental protocol, I was called out of the country. Instead of postponing the study, she managed to pull it off in one long evening with the help of the rest of our team.
5. See Brian Wansink, Robert J. Kent, and Stephen J. Hoch, "An

Anchoring and Adjustment Model of Purchase Quantity Decisions," *Journal of Marketing Research* 35:1 (February 1998): 71–81.

6. The speed at which you gain weight after going off a diet is almost always directly related to the speed you lost the weight to begin with. If you miraculously lose 10 pounds in two days with the new Celebrity Fad Diet, you're likely to miraculously gain it back almost as fast.

7. See Maureen T. Mcguire, Rena R. Wing, Mary L. Klem, and James O. Hill, "What Predicts Weight Regain in a Group of Successful Weight Losers?" *Journal of Consulting and Clinical Psychology* 67:2 (1999): 177–85.

8. Quotations were adapted from "Last-Minute Diet Secrets," *People* (March 16, 2004): 122–25.

9. This conclusion is from a series of studies alluded to in David A. Levitsky, "The Non-Regulation of Food Intake in Humans: Hope for Reversing the Epidemic of Obesity," *Physiology & Behavior* 86:5 (December 2005): 623–32.

10. Much of the best work on restrained eaters has been conducted by Janet Polivy and C. Peter Herman. A typical example of this is Janet Polivy, J. Coleman, and C. Peter Herman, "The Effect of Deprivation on Food Cravings and Eating Behavior in Restrained and Unrestrained Eaters," *International Journal of Eating Disorders* 38:4 (December 2005): 301–09.

11. This syndicated column was widely reprinted with the name of the nationally known psychologist. It was taken from "News of the Weird," *Funny Times* (October 2005): 25.

12. The best current thinking on this is being done by Roy Baumeister. See Roy F. Baumeister, "Yielding to Temptation: Self-Control Failure, Impulsive Purchasing, and Consumer Behavior," *Journal of Consumer Research* 28:4 (2002): 670–76. Other research includes that by Erica M. Okada, "Justification Effects on Consumer Choice of Hedonic and Utilitarian Goods," *Journal of Marketing Research* 42:1 (2005): 43–53; and by Baba Shiv and Alexander Fedorikhin, "Heart and Mind in

Conflict: The Interplay of Affect and Cognition in Consumer Decision Making," *Journal of Consumer Research* 26 (December 1999): 278–92.

13. N. E. Sherwood, Robert W. Jeffrey, Simone French, et al., "Predictors of Weight Gain in the Pound of Prevention Study," *International Journal of Obesity* 24:4 (April 2000): 395–403.

14. If you burn off the same number of calories each day as you eat, you are "in energy balance." The exact number of calories you need to be in energy balance varies depending on your weight and how much you move during the day. Smaller adults burn fewer calories a day than larger adults; active people more than inactive people.

15. A pound is roughly equivalent to 3,500 calories. Eating three Jelly Belly jelly beans a day (12 calories) would lead to 4,380 calories over the year. Similarly, drinking one can of Coca-Cola (139 calories) each day would amount to 101,470 calories—29 pounds—over a two-year period.

16. See James O. Hill and John C. Peters, "Environmental Contributions to the Obesity Epidemic," *Science,* 280 (5368): 1371–74.

17. See Bradley J. Willcox, M.D., D. Craig Willcox, Ph.D., and Makoto Suzuki, M.D., *The Okinawa Program* (New York: Clarkson Potter, 2001).

2. The Forgotten Food

1. People generally thought they ate about 28 percent less than they actually did. See Brian Wansink and Lawrence W. Linder, "Interactions Between Forms of Fat Consumption and Restaurant Bread Consumption," *International Journal of Obesity* 27:7 (2003): 866–68.

2. Two excellent research projects addressing this are David A. Booth and Richard P. J. Freeman, "Are Calories Attributed or

Sensed," *Appetite* 24:2 (April 1995): 184; and Michael R. Lowe, "Eating Motives and the Controversy Over Dieting: Eating Less Than Needed Versus Less Than Wanted," *Obesity Research* 13:5 (May 2005): 797–806.

3. Adapted from "No Expense Spared for Big Day of Fun," *USA Today* (February 4, 2005), E-2.

4. Brian Wansink and Collin R. Payne, "The Chicken-Bone Diet: Consumption Monitoring and Intake" (2006), under review. The study was filmed for ABC's *20/20* and the entertaining clips can be seen at www.MindlessEating.org.

5. The Prison Pounds Mystery is based on a conversation with Sarah Jo Brenner, a journalist from Urbana, Illinois.

6. This BMI formula works for countries like the United States and Guam, which still use the Imperial measurement system of feet and pounds. If you're from any of the 200+ countries using the metric system, your BMI is even easier to figure out. Take your height in meters, multiply it by itself, divide this number into your weight in kilos.

7. The Body Frame Rule of Thumb can be found in Diane Irons' interesting book *The World's Best Diet Secrets*.

8. Barbara Rolls, *The Volumetrics Eating Plan* (2005). Additional work on this topic of energy density has been conducted with Dr. Richard Mattes at Purdue University, Dr. Roland L. Weinsier at the University of Alabama at Birmingham, and Dr. Terry Brownlee at the Duke University Diet and Fitness Center. An interview with Dr. Rolls on this topic can be viewed in the ABC *20/20* episode on obesity mentioned in note 4 above.

9. Great diet ideas using this energy density approach can be found in Howard M. Shapiro, *Dr. Shapiro's Picture Perfect Weight Loss: The Visual Program for Permanent Weight Loss* (New York: Warner Books, Inc., 2000).

10. See S. C. Wooley, "Physiologic Versus Cognitive Factors in Short-Term Food Regulation in the Obese and Nonobese," *Psychosomatic Medicine* 34 (1972): 62–8.

11. See Rick Bell and Patti L. Pliner, "Time to Eat: The Relationship Between the Number of People Eating and Meal Duration in Three Lunch Settings," *Appetite* 41 (2003): 215–18.

12. See Brian Wansink, James E. Painter, and Jill North, "Bottomless Bowls: Why Visual Cues of Portion Size May Influence Intake," *Obesity Research* 13:1 (January 2005): 93–100.

13. See Brian Wansink, Collin R. Payne, Pierre Chandon, and Paul Rozin, "The French Paradox Redux: Internal and External Cues of Meal Cessation" (2006), under review.

14. This gap in our calorie estimation and the exaggerated gap among obese people has been widely reported by top scholars over the past 20 years. The classic studies include: David Lansky and Kelly D. Brownell, "Estimates of Food Quantity and Calories: Errors in Self-Report Among Obese Patients," *American Journal of Clinical Nutrition* 35:4 (1982): 727–32; M. Barbara, E. Livingstone, and Alison E. Black, "Markers of the Validity of Reported Energy Intake," *Journal of Nutrition* 133:3 (2003): 895S–920S. Janet A. Tooze, Amy F. Subar, Frances E. Thompson, Richard Troiano, Arthur Schatzkin, and Victor Kipnis, "Psychosocial Predictors of Energy Underreporting in a Large Doubly Labeled Water Study," *The American Journal of Clinical Nutrition* 79:5 (2004): 795–804.

15. See Shirley S. Wang, Kelly Brownell, and Thomas Wadden, "The Influence of the Stigma of Obesity on Overweight Individuals," *International Journal of Obesity* 28:10 (October 2004): 1333–37.

16. This is mathematically predicted by a compressive power function. The details (including the math) can be found in Pierre Chandon and Brian Wansink, "Obesity and the Calorie Underestimation Bias: A Psychophysical Model of Fast-Food Meal Size Estimation," *Journal of Marketing Research* (2007), forthcoming.

17. There are important implications for how diet counseling is conducted. See Brian Wansink and Pierre Chandon "Meal Size, Not Body Size, Explains Food Calorie Estimation Errors," *Annals*

of Internal Medicine (September 2006), forthcoming. Fortunately, we also found an easy way to de-bias calorie estimates. When people estimate the calories in each item of a meal (the calories in the chicken, in the corn, in the salad) and then add them up, they are usually within 5 to 10 percent of the correct number.

3. Surveying the Tablescape

1. This 92 percent figure pops up in our studies again and again. See Brian Wansink and Matthew M. Cheney, "Super Bowls: Serving Bowl Size and Food Consumption," *Journal of the American Medical Association* 293:14 (April 2005): 1727–28.
2. Much of this section's discussion on package size is based on the paper, Brian Wansink, "Can Package Size Accelerate Usage Volume?" *Journal of Marketing* 60:3 (July 1996): 1–14.
3. In a more carefully controlled lab study, the differences were 63 and 122 M&M's (see "Can Package Size Accelerate Usage Volume?"). For this reason, some people buy smaller packages even if they end up costing more per M&M. Similarly, people who are trying to quit smoking often buy single packs of cigarettes instead of the larger 10-pack cartons, which are often a third of the price.
4. This idea of consumption norms is set forth in Brian Wansink, "Environmental Factors That Increase the Food Intake and Consumption Volume of Unknowing Consumers," *Annual Review of Nutrition* 24 (2004): 455–79.
5. Different countries have different norms. For instance, Paul Rozin's work shows meals served in Chinese restaurants in Philadelphia are 72 percent heftier than those served in Chinese restaurants in Paris.
6. See Brian Wansink, "Can Package Size Accelerate Usage Volume?"
7. See Abby Ellin, "For Overweight Children, Are 'Fat Camps' a Solution?" *New York Times* on the web (June 2005).

8. See Brian Wansink and Koert van Ittersum, "Bottoms Up! The Influence of Elongation and Pouring on Consumption Volume," *Journal of Consumer Research* 30:3 (December 2003): 455–63.

9. Although we planned to collect the data as a team, that's not the way it worked. As *Philadelphia Inquirer* columnist Michael Klein pithily described in his New Year's Day column in 2006, "In the true academic tradition, Wansink said he had planned to send students into the field to do the legwork. 'But you can't send 19-year-olds into bars,' he said last week." I ended up having to do it myself, but I still use the word "we" to give credit to the team who helped plan the bartender portion of this study back in 1995.

10. Koert van Ittersum and I also took 198 college students and gave them 10 practice trials pouring the exact amount. When we changed the glasses, they, too, overpoured. These last two studies were published together in Brian Wansink and Koert van Ittersum, "Shape of Glass and Amount of Alcohol Poured: Comparative Study of Effect of Practice and Concentration," *British Medical Journal* 331 (2005): 1512–14.

11. See also Priya Raghubir and Aradhna Krishna, "Vital Dimensions in Volume Perception: Can the Eye Fool the Stomach?" *Journal of Marketing Research* 36:3 (1999): 313–26; and Valerie Folkes and S. Matta, "The Effect of Package Shape on Consumers' Judgments of Product Volume: Attention as a Mental Contaminant," *Journal of Consumer Research* 31:2 (September 2004): 390–401.

12. Straw drinkers also need to beware of big straws. Henry T. Lawless, Sharon Bender, Carol Oman, and Cathy Pelletier, "Gender, Age, Vessel Size, Cup vs. Straw Sipping, and Sequence Effects on Sip Volume," *Dysphagia* 18:3 (Summer 2003): 196–202.

13. See Brian Wansink, Koert van Ittersum, and James E. Painter, "Ice Cream Illusions: Bowl Size, Spoon Size, and Serving Size," *American Journal of Preventive Medicine* (September 2006).

14. This was conducted with one of the three sections of the Understanding Consumer Choice course I was teaching to

MBA students at the University of Illinois. Thanks to my 90-minute bowl-size intensive, this section rated my teacher evaluations for the course 8 percent lower than my other two sections. A small price to pay for a *JAMA* article.

15. See Brian Wansink and Matthew M. Cheney, "Super Bowls: Serving Bowl Size and Food Consumption," *Journal of the American Medical Association* 293:14 (April 2005): 1727–28.

16. Barbara J. Rolls, Edward A. Rowe, Edmund T. Rolls, Breda Kingston, Angela Megson, and Rachael Gunary, "Variety in a Meal Enhances Food Intake in Man," *Physiology and Behavior* 26 (1981): 215–21. David L. Katz and Catherine S. Katz, *Flavor Point Diet, The Delicious, Breakthrough Plan to Turn Off Your Hunger and Lose the Weight for Good* (Emmaus, PA: Rodale Books, 2005).

19. See J. Jeffrey Inman, "The Role of Sensory-Specific Satiety in Attribute-Level Variety Seeking," *Journal of Consumer Research* 28:1 (2001): 105–20.

18. See Edward T. Rolls and J. H. Rolls, "Olfactory Sensory-Specific Satiety in Humans," *Physiology and Behavior* 61 (1997): 461.

19. A variety of studies with more generalizable populations are reported in Barbara E. Kahn and Brian Wansink, "The Influence of Assortment Structure on Perceived Variety and Consumption Quantities," *Journal of Consumer Research* 30:4 (March 2004): 519–33. As with the bartender article, special thanks to David Mick, the editor, for helping these ideas come to life.

20. There are two explanations for this. First, the larger the number of food or flavors we believe we see, the more we imagine we'll enjoy it. The second reason is a bit more complicated. When it comes down to how much food we should take, we generally don't know how much we want. There aren't right and wrong answers. One thing we do is consider how much is normal or appropriate or typical to take and then we let that number guide us. For instance, when we see what appears to be a large variety of food or a large amount of food, we think

that it's normal and appropriate to take more. With the jelly beans, people estimated there were more flavors of jelly beans when they were mixed up, and this influenced what they took. They took what they thought was normal or appropriate.

21. The bowls with seven M&M's included green, orange, blue, yellow, brown, tan, and red; the bowls with ten also contained gold, pink, and teal. The details can be found in Barbara. E. Kahn and Brian Wansink, "The Influence of Assortment Structure on Perceived Variety and Consumption Quantities," *Journal of Consumer Research* 30: 4 (March 2004): 519–33.

22. The variety of an assortment can be mathematically determined and a useful tool for doing so can be found in Stephen J. Hoch, Eric L. Bradlow, and Brian Wansink, "The Variety of Assortment," *Marketing Science* 18:4 (1999): 527–46.

4. The Hidden Persuaders Around Us

1. The candy was given to secretaries who were located in out-of-the-way places where there wasn't much traffic and where there was little chance of their candy being pilfered by passers-by. See Brian Wansink, James E. Painter, and Yeon-Kyung Lee, "Proximity's Influence on Estimated and Actual Candy Consumption," *International Journal of Obesity* 30:5 (May 2006): 871–75.

2. Although this is a common science fair study, the original study conducted by Stanley Schachter showed the impact to be most relevant to obese people. Most replications of this study have shown the inconvenience of a wrapper influences nearly everyone.

3. It used to be thought that how hungry we felt could be predicted by small increasing contractions in our stomach. (When they become extreme we hear them as growls.) We now know that these contractions are not necessary for us to feel hunger.

4. See Jacques Le Magnen, *Neurobiology of Feeding and Nutrition* (New York: Academic Press, 1992). Alexandra W. Logue, *The Psychology of Eating and Drinking,* 3rd edition (New York: Brunner-Routledge, 2004). See also Peter J. Rogers and Andrew J. Hill, "Breakdown of Dietary Restraint Following Mere Exposure to Food Stimuli: Interrelationships Between Restraint, Hunger, Salivation, and Food Intake," *Addictive Behaviors* 14 (1989): 387–97.

5. See Brian Wansink and Rohit Deshpandé, " 'Out of Sight, Out of Mind': The Impact of Household Stockpiling on Usage Rates," *Marketing Letters* 5:1 (1994): 91–100.

6. See Phil McGraw, *The Ultimate Weight Solution: The 7 Keys to Weight Loss Freedom* (New York: Free Press, 2003).

7. See also Stanley Schachter and Judith Rodin, *Obese Humans and Rats* (New York: John Wiley & Sons, 1974). See also Stanley Schachter, "Some Extraordinary Facts About Obese Humans and Rats," *American Psychologist* 26 (1971): 129–44, and Patti Pliner, "Effect of External Cues on the Thinking Behavior of Obese and Normal Subjects," *Journal of Abnormal Psychology* 82 (1968): 233–38.

8. This study is one of Schachter's most clever in this area: Stanley L. Schachter, "Manipulated Time and Eating Behavior," *Journal of Personality and Social Psychology* 10 (1968): 98–106, and Harvey P. Weingarten, "Meal Initiation Controlled by Learned Cues: Basic Behavioral Properties," *Appetite* 5 (1984): 147–58.

9. The study where we gave people chocolates in their desks can be found in James E. Painter, Brian Wansink, and Julie B. Hieggelke, "How Visibility and Convenience Influence Candy Consumption," *Appetite* 38:3 (June 2002), 237–38. See also Brian Wansink, James E. Painter, and Yeon-Kyung Lee, "Proximity's Influence on Estimated and Actual Candy Consumption," *International Journal of Obesity* 30:5 (May 2006): 871–75.

10. This particular study focused on non-Asian diners at the two extremes of normal weight (BMI<25) and obese (BMI>30),

not on those who are overweight but not obese (BMI between 25 and 30). The Chopsticks study is part of a larger study: Brian Wansink and Collin R. Payne, "The Cues and Correlates of Overeating at the Chinese Buffet," Cornell University Food and Brand Lab working paper. Our undercover All-You-Can-Eat investigation of chopstick use is based on the comments made in Stanley Schachter, L. N. Friedman, and J. Handler, "Who Eats with Chopsticks?" in eds. S. Schachter and J. Rodin, *Obese Humans and Rats* (Hoboken, NJ: Wiley & Sons, 1974).

11. For more fascinating research on humans and rats, see David A. Levitsky, "Putting Behavior Back into Feeding Behavior: A Tribute to George Collier," *Appetite* 38 (2002): 143–8. See also Stanley Schachter and Judith Rodin, *Obese Humans and Rats.*

12. A bold proponent of field research with food is Herb Meiselman, co-editor of the journal *Food Quality and Preference.* This piece of research can be found in Herbert L. Meiselman, Duncan Hedderley, Sarah L. Staddon, Barry J. Pierson, and Catherine R. Symongs, "Effect of Effort on Meal Selection and Meal Acceptability in a Student Cafeteria," *Appetite* 23 (1994): 43–55.

13. See A. W. Meyers, A. J. Stunkard, and M. Coll, "Food Accessibility and Food Choice," *Archives of General Psychiatry,* 37:10 (October 1980), 1133–35.

14. See Brian Wansink, Armand Cardello, and Jill North, "Fluid Consumption and the Potential Role of Canteen Shape in Minimizing Dehydration," *Military Medicine* 170:10 (October 2005): 871–73.

15. In the late 1990s, we surveyed people about the foods they buy and never use. Many of the items they never used included those they bought in bulk for an event (such as a party) that never happened. See Brian Wansink, S. Adam Brasel, and Stephen Amjad, "The Mystery of the Cabinet Castaway: Why We Buy Products We Never Use," *Journal of Family and Consumer Science* 92:1 (2001): 104–08.

16. See Pierre Chandon and Brian Wansink, "When Are Stock-

piled Products Consumed Faster? A Convenience-Salience Framework of Post-Purchase Consumption Incidence and Quantity," *Journal of Marketing Research* 39:3 (August 2002): 321–35. Special thanks to Russ Winer (now dean at NYU), the editor who helped us shape this article and bring it to light.

5. Mindless Eating Scripts

1. We've investigated this in a number of qualitative and quantitative studies. One of the more interesting findings involved 150 Chicagoans and 150 Parisians who were asked to rate a series of statements about their eating behavior on a 1–9 scale (1 = disagree; 9 = agree). See Brian Wansink, Collin Payne, Pierre Chandon, and Paul Rozen, "The French Paradox Redux: The Influence of Internal and External Cues in Meal Cessation," under review.

2. See John M. DeCastro, "Eating Behavior: Lessons from the Real World of Humans," *Ingestive Behavior and Obesity* 16 (2000): 800–13; and John M. DeCastro, "Family and Friends Produce Greater Social Facilitation of Food-Intake Than Other Companions," *Physiology and Behavior* 56 (1994): 445–55.

3. See C. Peter Herman, Deborah A. Roth, and Janet Polivy, "Effects of the Presence of Others on Food Intake: A Normative Interpretation," *Psychological Bulletin* 129:6 (November 2003): 873–86.

4. See Rick Bell and Patti L. Pliner, "Time to Eat: The Relationship Between the Number of People Eating and Meal Duration in Three Lunch Settings," *Appetite* 41 (2003): 215–18.

5. See Shelley Chaiken and Patti L. Pliner, "Eating, Social Motives, and Self-Presentation in Women and Men," *Journal of Experimental Social Psychology* 26 (1990): 240–54.

6. See Brian Wansink, Collin R. Payne, Se-Bum Park, and

Junyong Kim, "I Am How Much I Eat: How Self-Monitoring Influences Food Intake on Dates," under review.

7. Although it is frequently found that television viewing, food intake, and obesity are related, these correlational studies are often confounded with factors such as a general lack of physical activity. Nevertheless, they do suggest an important relationship between distracted activity and consumption intake.

8. A number of researchers have shown correlational results between TV viewing and weight. These include David A. Crawford, Robert W. Jeffery, and Simone A. French, "Television Viewing, Physical Inactivity and Obesity," *International Journal of Obesity* 23:4 (April 1999): 427–40; Natalie Stroebele and John M. DeCastro, "Television Viewing Is Associated with an Increase in Meal Frequency in Humans," *Appetite* 42:1 (February 2004): 111–13.

9. This is from the provocatively titled working paper by Natalie Stroebele and John M. DeCastro, "Television Viewing Nearly Adds an Additional Meal to Daily Intake," manuscript under review.

10. Distractions such as television, reading, movies, and sporting events may simply redirect attention to the point where orosensory signals of satiation are ignored.

11. The poll was commissioned by the American Dietetic Association ConAgra Foods Fundation Home Food Safety program. It was reported in a *USA Today* article by Nanci Hellmich, October 1, 2004, p. 8D.

12. See France Bellisle and Anne-Marie Dalix, "Cognitive Restraint Can Be Offset by Distraction, Leading to Increased Meal Intake in Women," *American Journal of Clinical Nutrition* 74 (2001): 197–200.

13. The sample size of this study will be somewhat of a shocker. What needs to be realized is that it was published in a highly regarded academic journal. Here goes. This study involved only two amnesiac patients. One started eating the second

meal only 10 minutes after the first and the other ate it 30 minutes after. A great read at Paul Rozin, Sara Dow, Morris Moscovitch, and Suparna Rajaram, "What Causes Humans to Begin and End a Meal? A Role for Memory for What Has Been Eaten, as Evidenced by a Study of Multiple Meal Eating in Amnesic Patients," *Psychological Science* 9 (1998): 392–96.

14. Stanley L. Schachter, "Manipulated Time and Eating Behavior," *Journal of Personality and Social Psychology* 10 (1968): 98–106; Harvey P. Weingarten, "Meal Initiation Controlled by Learned Cues: Basic Behavioral Properties," *Appetite* 5 (1984): 147–58, and Judith Rodin, "Effects of Distraction on the Performance of Obese and Normal Subjects," in ed., S. Schachter and J. Rodin, *Obese Humans and Rats* (New York: Wiley & Sons, 1974).

15. Although this is a short, simple paper, it's one of those I seem to bring up in casual conversation quite a bit: Ronald E. Milliman, "The Influence of Background Music on the Behavior of Restaurant Patrons," *Journal of Consumer Research* 13:1 (1986): 286–89.

16. See Joseph G. Lavin and Harry T. Lawless, "Effects of Color and Odor on Judgments of Sweetness Among Children and Adults," *Food Quality and Preference* 9 (1998): 283.

17. Thanks to the cooperation of the manager and staff at the Hardee's restaurant (now a Carl's Jr. restaurant) at 1614 Neil Street in Champaign, Illinois).

18. Two thousand miles away from the Monell Center are Dr. Alan Hirsch's labs in Chicago. His labs have provided preliminary evidence that the types of smells we're attracted to may be related partly to our personalities. See Alan Hirsch, *What Flavor Is Your Personality? Discover Who You Are by Looking at What You Eat* (Naperville, IL: Sourcebooks, Inc., 2001).

19. This is only the tip of the sensory iceberg when it comes to the great sensory work done at Monell: Julie A. Mennella and Gary K. Beauchamp, "The Early Development of Human Flavor Preferences," in ed. Elizabeth D. Capaldi, *Why We Eat*

What We Eat: The Psychology of Eating (Washington, D.C.: American Psychological Association, 1996).

20. www.cinnabon.com on February 17, 2006.

21. A bit more background on the sensory differences in the field versus the lab can be found in Caas de Graaf, Armand V. Cardello, F. Matthew Kramer, Larry L. Lesher, Herbert L. Meiselman, and Howard G. Schutz, "A Comparison Between Liking Ratings Obtained Under Laboratory and Field Conditions: The Role of Choice," *Appetite* 44:1 (February 2005): 15–22.

22. See Diane Irons, *The World's Best-Kept Diet Secrets: Lose Weight Quickly, Safely, and Permanently* (Naperville, IL: Sourcebooks, Inc., 1998).

23. This temperature theory of hunger was first proposed in the 1940s: John. R. Brobeck, "Food Intake as a Mechanism of Temperature Regulation," *Journal of Biology and Medicine* 20 (1948): 545–52.

24. This is one reason why people who live around the equator tend to be thin and also why their food is so much spicier than up in Lapland or in Medicine Hat, Canada. When the weather is hot, spicy food stimulates our stomach and makes us want to eat more. It also makes us want to drink more liquids.

25. Storm spots are one example of situation-specific suggestions. The power of such suggestions were the basis of dissertation that is summarized in Brian Wansink and Michael L. Ray, "Advertising Strategies to Increase Usage Frequency," *Journal of Marketing* 60:1 (January 1996): 31–46.

6. The Name Game

1. Scientifically speaking, our taste is objective, but our interpretation of what we taste is subjective. We can't trick our taste buds, but we can trick what we *think* our taste buds taste.

2. See Heli M. Tuorila, Herbert L. Meiselman, Armand V.

Cardello, and Larry L. Lesher, "Effect of Expectations and the Definition of Product Category on Acceptance of Unfamiliar Foods," *Food Quality and Preference* 9:6 (1998): 421–30.

3. This pretest paved the way for a larger-scale study involving lemon and chocolate yogurt served in dark rooms with conflicting scents. See Brian Wansink, Alan O. Wright, and Collin R. Payne, "Olfactory Suggestiveness and Evaluation," working paper.

4. In 2001, the Lab did a large-scale quantitative survey on how World War II influenced food habits of Americans who were involved in the war. Billy was one of the veterans who completed the survey, and he included this handwritten story. More on our World War II study can be found in Chapter 8.

5. See Brian Wansink, Collin R. Payne, James E. Painter, and Jill North, "What Is Beautiful Tastes Good: Visual Cues and Taste Evaluation," *Food Quality and Preference,* under review.

6. Nothing gives a better appreciation of the theater that occurs in the kitchen of a world-class restaurant than Anthony Bourdain's irreverent classic *Kitchen Confidential: Adventures in the Culinary Underbelly* (New York: Ecco Press, HarperCollins, 2000).

7. This is an example of a piece of research where the results inadvertently leaked out to restaurant and hospitality industry magazines long before the study was actually published. I was surprised when I was giving a talk at a culinary institute in Florence in the spring of 2004 and saw it on a reading list, sans the names of my co-authors and me. The official version is Brian Wansink, Koert van Ittersum, and James E. Painter, "How Descriptive Food Names Bias Sensory Perceptions in Restaurants," *Food Quality and Preference* 16:5 (2005): 393–400.

8. See Brian Wansink, James E. Painter, and Koert van Ittersum, "Descriptive Menu Labels' Effect on Sales," *Cornell Hotel and Restaurant Administrative Quarterly* 42:6 (December 2001): 68–72.

9. These are the February 13, 2006 menus downloaded from the websites of the two schools. In addition to the items listed for Phillips Exeter Academy, their menu also had grilled chicken breast, cole slaw, and gingerbread with topping. In 1996, the Latin inscription over the main entrance to the Academy Building was changed to a more gender-inclusive version *"Hic quaerite pueri puellaeque virtutem et scientiam."*

10. See Graham Lawton, "Angelic Host," *New Scientist* 184 (December 2004): 68–69.

11. See Ralph I. Allison and Kenneth P. Uhl, "Influence of Beer Brand Identification on Taste Perception," *Journal of Marketing Research* 1 (August 1964): 36–39.

12. The World War II homefront enlisted all sorts of people— including social scientists—to help move through those troubled times. For a little taste of drama: Brian Wansink, "Changing Eating Habits on the Home Front: Lost Lessons from World War II Research," *Journal of Public Policy and Marketing* 21:1 (Spring 2002): 90–99. Special thanks to Connie Pechmann for helping these ideas come to light.

13. While the National Soybean Research Center initiated these early projects with soy, financial support for these studies also came from the Council for Agricultural Research, the Illinois Soybean Program Operating Board, and the Illinois Center for Soy Foods.

14. Russians have a different problem. In Russian, the word "soy" sounds like an acronym for a common nuclear bomb system. The best overview of these association studies is: Brian Wansink, *Marketing Nutrition: Soy, Functional Foods, Biotechnology, and Obesity* (Champaign: University of Illinois Press, 2005); Brian Wansink and Randall Westgren, "Profiling Taste-Motivated Segments," *Appetite* 4:3 (December 2003): 323–27; Brian Wansink, "Overcoming the Taste Stigma of Soy," *Journal of Food Science* 68:8 (September 2003): 2604–06.

15. This did not happen with everyone, however. People who had classified themselves as being very health conscious were

uninfluenced by the soy label. That is, having "soy" on the label didn't hurt their evaluation, but it also didn't help it any. It simply had no effect. More can be found in Brian Wansink and Se-Bum Park, "Sensory Suggestiveness and Labeling: Do Soy Labels Bias Taste?" *Journal of Sensory Studies* 17:5 (November 2002): 483–91.

7. In the Mood for Comfort Food

1. See Brian Wansink, Matthew M. Cheney, and Nina Chan, "Exploring Comfort Food Preferences Across Gender and Age," *Physiology and Behavior* 79:4 (2003): 739–47.
2. This basic bad mood/bad food–good mood/good food relationship has been explored in a number of papers currently under review at academic journals: Laurette Dube, Jordan L. LeBel, and J. Lu, "Affect Asymmetry and Comfort Food Consumption;" and Brian Wansink and Collin Payne, "Do You Binge-Eat When You Are Happy? The Effects of Mood on Comfort Food Consumption."
3. Two manuscripts that explore the general theory behind this using controlled lab studies are Nitika Garg, Brian Wansink, and J. Jeffrey Inman, "The Influence of Incidental Affect on Consumer's Food Intake" (2007), forthcoming at *Journal of Marketing,* and Brian Wansink, Meryl P. Gardner, Junyong Kim, and Se-Bum Park, "Comfort Food, Mood, and Intake," under review.
4. The original description of how to do laddering can be found in Thomas J. Reynolds and Jonathan Gutman, "Laddering Theory, Method, Analysis, and Interpretation," *Journal of Advertising Research* (February/March 1988): 11–31. Since this time, the method has been modified to better suit different contexts, such as foods or high-equity brands: Brian Wansink, "Using Laddering to Understand and Leverage a Brand's Equity," *Qualitative Market Research* 6:2 (2003): 111–18. See also Brian

Wansink, "New Techniques to Generate Key Marketing Insights," *Marketing Research* (Summer 2000): 28–36.

5. This area of food identification is fascinating and is tackled by a number of different methods. A few novel ones include Carol Bisogni, Mark Connors, Carol M. Devine, and Jeffrey Sobal, "Who We Are and How We Eat: A Qualitative Study of Identities in Food Choice," *Journal of Nutrition Education and Behavior* 34:3 (May–June 2002): 128–39; and Michael W. Lynn and Judy Harris, "Individual Differences in the Pursuit of Uniqueness Through Consumption," *Journal of Applied Social Psychology* 27 (1997): 1861–83.

6. The primary purpose of this project was to develop a new statistical technique. The soup predictions were simply a way to test it. See Brian Wansink and SeaBum Park, "Accounting for Taste: Prototypes that Predict Preference," *Journal of Database Marketing,* 7:4, (2000), 308–20.

7. See Brian Wansink, Steven Sonka, Peter Goldsmith, Jorge Chiriboga, and Nilgun Eren, "Increasing the Acceptance of Soy-Based Foods," *Journal of International Food and Agribusiness Marketing* 17:1 (2005): 33–55.

8. I've also wondered how many of these people are Apple computer users. At one point, this short two-page article in *American Demographics* was the most frequently downloaded article on the www.ConsumerPsychology.com website. See Brian Wansink and Cynthia Sangerman, "Engineering Comfort Foods," *American Demographics* (July 2000): 66–7.

9. See Brian Wansink and Cynthia Huffman, "A Framework for Revitalizing Mature Brands," *Journal of Brand and Product Management* 10:4 (2001): 228–42.

10. Adapted in part from Doris Wild Helmering and Dianne Hales, *Think Thin, Be Thin* (New York: Broadway Books, 2004): 77.

11. See Brian Wansink, Koert van Ittersum, and Carolina Werle, "How Combat Influences Unfamiliar Food Preferences: Do Marines Eat Japanese Food?", under review. Bad associations

from World War II also influence attitudes toward German foods, one reason why Swanson's TV dinner "Sauerbraten-Bavarian Red Cabbage-Spaetzle" was thought to have flopped in the late 1950s.

12. In reality, the fact that a study comes out differently than planned is nothing new to us. In some cases, we make mistakes, like using tube-clogging chicken noodle soup in our Refillable Bowl study. In other cases, accidents happen, like when someone knocks a $1,400 wireless scale off a table. In still other contexts, our study design is just not clever enough to give us a clear answer. That's why we do so many things a second and third time.

8. Nutritional Gatekeepers

1. See Brian Wansink and Keong-mi Lee, "Cooking Habits Provide a Key to 5 a Day Success," *Journal of the American Dietetic Assocation* 104:11 (November 2004): 1648–50.

2. See Brian Wansink, "Focus on Nutritional Gatekeepers and the 72% Solution," *Journal of the American Dietetic Association,* (September 2006), in press. Interestingly, we've repeated this with a lot of different people. Good cooks, non-cooks, young parents, empty nesters, grandmothers, single moms. They vary a little bit, but all end up estimating right around 72 percent.

3. See Brian Wansink, "Profiling Nutritional Gatekeepers: Three Methods for Differentiating Influential Cooks," *Food Quality and Preference* 14:4 (June 2003): 289–97.

4. See Brian Wansink and Randall Westgren, "Profiling Taste-Motivated Segments," *Appetite* 41:3 (December 2003): 323–27; Brian Wansink and JaeHak Cheong, "Taste Profiles that Correlate with Soy Consumption in Developing Countries," *Pakistan Journal of Nutrition* 1:6 (December 2002): 276–78; and Brian Wansink and Keong-mi Lee, "Cooking Habits Provide a Key to 5 a Day Success."

5. When the first Nutritional Gatekeeper study was published, our reviewers wanted us to focus on methodology, not percentages. See Brian Wansink, "Profiling Nutritional Gatekeepers: Three Methods for Differentiating Influential Cooks," *Food Quality and Preference* 14:4 (June 2003): 289–97. The percentages appear in Brian Wansink, *Marketing Nutrition: Soy, Functional Foods, Biotechnology, and Obesity* (Champaign: University of Illinois Press, 2005).

6. Brian Wansink, Ganaël Bascoul, and Gary T. Chen, "The Sweet Tooth Hypothesis: How Fruit Consumption Relates to Snack Consumption," *Appetite,* 31:2 (June 2006), in press.

7. Picky eater at home? Take heart. Gentle persistence will be rewarded. One taste doesn't change a person. Professor Leann Birch has shown that it can take up to 15 one-bite attempts, but most children eventually come around to liking more than just french fries, ice cream, and Jell-O.

8. This longitudinal study involves control groups, panel diaries, and reliability checks, all of which are too boring for a sidebar. While anchovies (fresh, not cured) might be extreme, rest assured that my daughter, Audrey, isn't the only one in the study who is eating and enjoying them. Also, it's important to avoid foods that could cause choking, such as popcorn, nuts, potato chips, whole-kernel corn, berries, grapes, hot dogs, raw vegetables, raisins, and dry flake cereals. To keep abreast of the findings from this panel study, stay tuned to www.MindlessEating.org.

9. See Julie A. Mennella and Gary K. Beauchamp, "The Early Development of Human Flavor Preferences" in ed. Elizabeth D. Capaldi, *Why We Eat What We Eat: The Psychology of Eating* (Washington, D.C.: American Psychological Association, 1996).

10. This is a classic: Sibylle K. Escalona, "Feeding Disturbances in Very Young Children," *American Journal of Orthopsychiatry* 15 (1945): 76–80.

11. See T. M. Field, R. Woodson, R. Greenberg, and D. Cohen, "Discrimination and Imitation of Facial Expressions by Neonates," *Science* 218 (1982): 179–81.

12. Thanks to Alexandra Logue for this example from her inspiring book, *The Psychology of Eating and Drinking,* 3rd edition (New York: Brunner-Routledge, 2005).

13. See F. Baeyens, D. Vansteenwegen, J. De Houwer, and G. Crombex, "Observational Conditioning of Food Valence in Humans," *Appetite* 27 (1996): 235–50.

14. Much of the most interesting research in this area is by Leann L. Birch. See "Generalization of a Modified Food Preference," *Child Development* 52 (1981): 755–58.

15. See Kathleen M. Pike and Judith Rodin, "Mothers, Daughters, and Disordered Eating," *Journal of Abnormal Psychology,* 100 (1991): 198–204.

16. Exerpted from the American Dietetic Association's *Dieting for Dummies* (Hoboken, NJ: Wiley & Sons, 2004).

17. An excellent review of this research can be found in Alexandra Logue, *The Psychology of Eating and Drinking,* 3rd edition (New York: Brunner-Routledge, 2005).

18. This new area of study is focusing on why some children develop positive views toward healthy foods, while others don't. The foundation for this is based on what we learned about how comfort foods are formed with adults, which is found in Brian Wansink and Cynthia Sangerman, "Engineering Comfort Foods," *American Demographics* (July 2000): 66–67.

19. Both of these children, whose parents were originally from mainland China, were raised almost exclusively on Chinese food. Although iodine prevents thyroid conditions, this knowledge certainly wouldn't encourage increased seaweed consumption among four-year-olds.

20. From Carolyn Wyman's very entertaining book, *Better Than Homemade* (Philadelphia: Quirk Books, 2004).

21. In France, this is a common perception of snacking. Among the bourgeoisie, snacking between meals is still considered a behavior well-mannered people don't do.

22. Many of these classic studies were conducted at the Child

Behavior Labs, when both Birch and Fisher were at the University of Illinois at Urbana-Champaign. Leann L. Birch and Jennifer O. Fisher, "Mother's Child-Feeding Practices Influence Daughters' Eating and Weight," *American Journal of Clinical Nutrition* 71 (2000): 1054–61; Leann L. Birch, Linda McPhee, B. C. Shoba, Lois Steinberg, and Ruth Krehbiel, "Clean Up Your Plate: Effects of Child Feeding Practices on the Conditioning of Meal Size," *Learning and Motivation* 18 (1987): 301–17. See also Jennifer O. Fisher, Barbara J. Rolls, and Leann L. Birch, "Children's Bite Size and Intake of an Entrée Are Greater with Large Portions Than with Age-Appropriate or Self-Selected Portions," *American Journal of Clinical Nutrition* 77 (2003): 1164–70.

23. The Idaho Plate Method was adapted from a Swedish meal-planning method by a group of Idaho dietitians. It works by visualizing how much space each of the major food groups should occupy on one plate. Details of how it varies across meals can be found at www.platemethod.com. At lunch and dinner, food should be portioned out so that one-fourth of the plate is covered with a starchy food (such as pasta, rice, or potatoes), one-fourth should have a protein or a meat source, and half should be filled with low-calorie "nonstarchy" vegetables (not potatoes, corn, or peas). To the side of the plate, there should be either one cup of milk or yogurt or a half cup of pudding or ice cream, as well as one small piece of fruit. The approach is not only easy to use, but also works well when eating outside the home, such as in a restaurant or at a family gathering. See H. Rizor, M. Smith, K. Thomas, J. Harker, and M. Rich, "Practical Nutrition: The Idaho Plate Method," *Practical Diabetology* 17 (1998): 42–45.

9. Fast-Food Fever

1. In 2005, the FDA charged the Keystone Group to develop a position paper for nutrition and labeling of away-from-home foods—fast food being a big piece of this. That's how I met Eric Haviland and that's the context in which he made this quote (December 14, 2005).

2. Fast food is also very predictable. There are no bad tables, bad waiters, or bad french fries.

3. Adapted from NPD Group, *Summary of Food Trends—2002* (2003), www.npd.com.

4. At the 2003 Food Forum hearing on packaging and portion sizes, Barbara J. Rolls and I were two of the primary academic speakers.

5. See Brian Wansink, Collin R. Payne, Pierre Chandon, and Jill North, "The McSubway Illusion: Health Halos and Biased Lunches," under review.

6. Okay, the definition of a calorie (which is 1/1000 of a "real" calorie, also known as a kilocalorie or kCal) is the amount of energy it takes to raise the temperature of 1 gram of water 1 degree Celsius. Let's assume your ice-cold beverage is 0 degrees Celsius, and your body is 37 degrees Celsius. Since there are 29.54 grams of water in an ounce, it will take 1,092 calories to heat up that ounce of water to your body temperature. This translates into about 1.1 kCal per ounce.

7. Estimate based on a marketplace survey of the 14 brands of granola that offer both low-fat and regular versions.

8. For both the granola and the chocolate studies, see Brian Wansink and Pierre Chandon, "Do Low Fat Nutrition Labels Lead to Obesity?" *Journal of Marketing Research* (2006), forthcoming.

9. The American Dietetic Association believes this is a big enough issue to have developed a position paper on it. See

Brian Wansink, "Position of the American Dietetic Association: Food and Nutrition Misinformation," *Journal of the American Dietetic Association,* 106 (2006): 601–7.

10. See Brian Wansink, Steven T. Sonka, Clare M. Hasler, "Front-Label Health Claims: When Less Is More," *Food Policy* 29:6 (December 2004) 659–67. In the lab-study version of this experiment (the version we published), we found that having "soy" on the package was enough to make them expect the taste to be terrible, and their taste buds obediently followed their expectations. See Brian Wansink and Se-Bum Park, "Sensory Suggestiveness and Labeling: Do Soy Labels Bias Taste?" *Journal of Sensory Studies* 17:5 (November 2002): 483–91.

11. Functional foods have properties that might reduce the risk of certain diseases. A full description of them and how consumers respond to them can be found in Brian Wansink, *Marketing Nutrition: Soy, Functional Foods, Biotechnology, and Obesity* (Champaign: University of Illinois Press, 2005).

12. A legion of great researchers have tackled this topic. For a sampling, see Christine Moorman, "A Quasi-Experiment to Assess the Consumer and Informational Determinants of Nutritional Information Processing Activities: The Case of the Nutrition Labeling and Education Act," *Journal of Public Policy & Marketing* 15 (Spring 1996): 28–44. J. Craig Andrews, Richard G. Netemeyer, and Scott Burton, "Consumer Generalization of Nutrient Content Claims in Advertising," *Journal of Marketing* 62:4 (1998): 62–75; Siva K. Balasubramanian and Catherine Cole, "Consumers' Search and Use of Nutrition Information: The Challenge and Promise of the Nutrition Labeling and Education Act," *Journal of Marketing* 66:3 (2002): 112; Christine Moorman, Kristin Diehl, David Brinberg, and Blair Kidwell, "Subjective Knowledge, Search Location and Consumer Choice," *Journal of Consumer Research* 31 (December 2004): 673–80.

13. See Brian Wansink, "How Do Front and Back Package Labels Influence Beliefs About Health Claims?" *Journal of Consumer*

Affairs 37:2 (Winter 2003): 305–16. Brian Wansink, "Overcoming the Taste Stigma of Soy," *Journal of Food Science* 68:8 (September 2003): 2604–06.

14. NPD Group 2003.

15. This positive win-win perspective has been gaining political momentum and this spirit of cooperation was an important subtheme of the National Governors' Association meeting in 2005–2006, which was chaired by Governor Mike Huckabee of Arkansas. See Brian Wansink and Mike Huckabee, "De-Marketing Obesity," *California Management Review* 47:4 (Summer 2005): 6–18.

16. See Lisa R. Young, *The Portion Teller* (New York: Broadway Books, 2005). Also see Lisa R. Young and Marion Nestle, "The Contribution of Expanding Portion Sizes to the US Obesity Epidemic," *American Journal of Public Health* 92 (2002): 246–49.

17. One question I'm often asked is, "Why do restaurants supersize in America more than in other countries?" I think this is largely because of the competition between chain restaurants. All the chains advertise, and to most people they're not tremendously differentiated (there are very subtle differences between Applebee's, Charlie's, Chili's, and so on). As long as they all seem to provide a "good value," they'll all get some of our business. As chain restaurants expand abroad, this phenomenon is almost sure to follow.

18. See Carolyn Wyman, *Better Than Homemade* (Philadelphia: Quirk Books, 2004).

19. When it comes to indulgent or "hedonic" products, we're much less price-sensitive than we are with daily items. It's one reason we buy our paper towels at Wal-Mart, but not perfume. This distinction in price-sensitivity is underscored in Pierre Chandon, Brian Wansink, and Gilles Laurent, "A Benefit Congruency Framework of Sales Promotion Effectiveness," *Journal of Marketing* 64:4 (October 2000): 65–81.

10. Mindlessly Eating Better

1. We're blessed with an embarrassment of food. It's easy to forget that less than 100 years ago, much of Eastern and Western Europe was starving. The widely acclaimed "heroic engineer" of European food aid and recovery after World War I actually *had been* an engineer—Herbert Hoover. And he'd also been a hungry nine-year-old orphan. For over 20 years, I've regularly visited his birthplace (and Presidential Library) in West Branch, Iowa. It's even where I proposed to my wife. While making a documentary in March of 2006, the veteran PBS producer Tom Spain told me, "You're probably the only person who gets choked up when he talks about Herbert Hoover . . . other than those who speak Dutch, German, or Russian."

2. There are a number of excellent books by good friends and premier scholars in this area, including: Kelly D. Brownell and Katherine Battle-Horgen, *Food Fight: The Inside Story of the Food Industry, America's Obesity Crisis and What We Can Do About It* (New York: The McGraw-Hill Companies, Inc., 2004); Marion Nestle, *Food Politics: How the Food Industry Influences Nutrition and Health* (Berkeley and Los Angeles: University of California Press, 2002). A compellingly crafted book regarding more general scientific pressures in the food industry is Robin Mather's *A Garden of Unearthly Delights: Bioengineering and the Future of Food* (New York: Dutton, published by the Penguin Group, 1995).

3. See James O. Hill, John C. Peters, Bonnie T. Jortberg, Pamela Peeke, *The Step Diet : Count Steps, Not Calories to Lose Weight and Keep It Off Forever* (New York: Workman Publishing, 2004). See also Simone A. French, Mary Story, Jayne A. Fulkerson, and Anne F. Gerlach, "Food Environment in Secondary Schools: À la Carte, Vending Machines, and Food Policies and Practices," *American Journal of Public Health* 93:7 (July 2003): 1161–67.

4. There are at least four other food-focused books in this area I think are top-level: Charles Stuart Platkin, *The Automatic Diet: The Proven 10-Step Process for Breaking Your Fat Pattern* (New York: Hudson Street Press, 2005); James M. Ferguson and Cassandra Ferguson, *Habits Not Diets: The Secret to Lifetime Weight Control* (Boulder, CO: Bull Publishing Company, 2003). Other books that balance both food and activity are Edward Abramson's *Body Intelligence: Lose Weight, Keep It Off, and Feel Great About Your Body Without Dieting* (New York: McGraw-Hill, 2005) and Jill Fleming's *Thin People Don't Clean Their Plates: Simple Lifestyle Choices for Permanent Weight Loss* (LaCrosse, WI: Inspiration Presentations Press, 2005).

5. See Dennis Bier, "Bringing National Policy to the Local Level: Building a Community Consensus on Health Disparities and How to Address Them," *Journal of Intellectual Disability Research* 48:4 (June 2004): 340; Laverne A. Berkel, Walker S.C. Poston, Rebecca S. Reeves, and John P. Foreyt, "Behavioral Interventions for Obesity," *Journal of the American Dietetic Association* 105:5 (May 2005): S35–S43.

6. Because of the relevance of my research to dieticians, I've been honored to be an affiliated member of the American Dietetic Association, even though I'm not a registered dietician.

7. A well-crafted personalized set of ideas can be found in Cathy Nonas' *Outwit Your Weight: Fat-Proof Your Life with More than 200 Tips, Tools, & Techniques to Help You Defeat Your Diet Danger Zones* (Emmaus, PA: Rodale, 2002).

8. If you need some ideas to get your creativity flowing, Appendix B gives five composite profiles of people who faced each of these diet danger zones, and it suggests some of the 100-calorie changes you could consider making with minimal interruption in your life.

9. You could ask a spouse or a good friend to keep you on track by asking if you've successfully completed your three changes that day. But that's not good either. First, it's not fair to your spouse or friend to have the burden of remembering. Second,

after the third day, even the most gentle reminders would sound like nagging.

10. The five diet danger zones that come up most frequently in our surveys are 1) meal stuffing, 2) snack grazing, 3) party binging, 4) restaurant indulging, and 5) desktop or dashboard dining. It's important to generate the ideas that you think are most easy and do-able.

11. An inspiring testimony by a very inspiring man is the step-by-step road to 100 pounds of weight loss by Mike Huckabee, *Quit Digging Your Grave with a Knife and Fork: A 12-Stop Program to End Bad Habits and Begin a Healthy Lifestyle* (New York: Center Street, 2005).

Acknowledgments

The studies in this book are ones I have conducted over the past twenty years. They have been generously supported by some of the greatest research universities and institutes in the United States and abroad, including Stanford, Dartmouth, Vrije Universiteit (Amsterdam), the Wharton School at the University of Pennsylvania, the University of Illinois at Urbana-Champaign, the U.S. Army Labs (Natick, MA), INSEAD (Fontainebleau, France), and Cornell University.

At this point, however, the greatest thanks needs to go to the College of Business at the University of Illinois for their belief in this research and their support of the bulk of it. Not all research studies are successful, and their support of my successful studies—and my unsuccessful ones—was critical in letting me help keep the Lab focused on our nutrition mission.

Academics is one of the world's greatest jobs because of the unbelievable people, like my past, current, and future co-authors. A partial list includes Michael Ray, Steve Hoch, Pierre Chandon, Rohit Deshpandé, Eric Bradlow, Barbara

Kahn, Bob Kent, Steve Sonka, Joost Pennings, Se-Bum Park, Adam Brasel, Jim Painter, Koert van Ittersum, Randy Westgren, Jill North, Junyong Kim, Matt Cheney, Armand Cardello, Mike Huckabee, Glenn Cordua, Collin Payne, Paul Rozin, Andrew Geier, John Peters, Lenny Vartanian, David Just, Jeff Sobel, Carolina Werle, and Peter Todd. This list also includes Sandra Cuellar, Pam Staub, Deb Gibbs, Marti Auler, and the Assistant Directors of the Food and Brand Lab over the years, including John Murray, Jorge Chirbogi, Mike Edmonds, Ron Wetzel, Erik Thorsen, Levi Bowman, Eduardo Baez, and Karla Monhke.

My special thanks to nurturers and supporters of me and of my vision of how food can transform lives: John Paxton, Bob Ridings, Michael Cheney, Michael Ray, Wendy Kleckner, Seenu Srinivasan, Jerry Blum, Steve Hoch, Julie Lee, Gary Bamossy, Kent Monroe, Huseyin Leblebici, Herb Meiselman, Bill Lesser, Ed McLaughlin, Susan Henry, Jay Walker, and John Dyson.

Much of my professional inspiration is from scholars who I believe are changing the food world. In my salad days, I hung on the inspiring words and ideas of Paul Rozin, Alexandra Logue, Peter Herman, Barbara Rolls, Leann Birch, Jim Hill, Kelly Brownell, Marion Nestle, Denny Bier, John Foreyt, Judith Stern, Charles Platkin, Elliot Blass, Rena Wing, John Peters, and Simone French, among others. More recently they have included my colleagues John Erdman, Bill Schultze, Chris Barrett, Cal Turvey, Harry Kaiser, John Cauley, David Levitsky, Jeff Sobal, Carol Devine, David Pelletier, Chris Olsen, and Jamie Dollohite.

Thanks to the tired eyes of Craig Wansink, John

Wansink, Matt Cheney, and Collin Payne for their detailed comments and advice on the book and to Bob Stein for incisive comments and advice as my attorney.

There are a handful of critical days in a person's life that dramatically alter its course. Some of these days are obvious to us when they happen, such as births and marriages, but I believe most of them aren't. They come, they go, we're changed, but don't know. My special thanks to all of those I'll never know who were there when they were most needed.

My special thanks to Toni Burbank, my editor at Bantam Dell, for tracking me down during my sabbatical in Fontainebleau, convincing me to write a popular book on my food research, and helping to gracefully lift this off the ground. Last, thanks to Jennifer and Audrey. See you at dinner.

Index

About the Author

An Iowa native, Brian Wansink (Ph.D., Stanford, 1990) is the John S. Dyson Professor of Marketing and Nutritional Science in the Applied Economics and Management Department at Cornell University, where he is Director of the Cornell Food and Brand Lab (www.FoodPsychology.Cornell. edu). Prior to Cornell, he was a professor at Dartmouth College, the Vrije Universiteit (The Netherlands), the Wharton School at the University of Pennsylvania, the University of Illinois at Urbana-Champaign, INSEAD (France), and a visiting scientist at the Natick Army Research Labs.

He is a Fulbright Senior Specialist in food marketing and nutrition, and he is the author of the books *Marketing Nutrition, Asking Questions,* and *Consumer Panels.* His award-winning academic research on food has been published in the world's top marketing, medical, and nutrition journals. It has been presented, translated, reported, and featured in television documentaries on every continent but Antarctica.

He lives with his family in Ithaca, New York, where he's a mediocre saxophone player in a rock-and-roll band and where he regularly enjoys both French food and french fries.

Share Your
Mindless Eating Secrets and Stories

What changes are you making to trim down your mindless margin? Share your ideas, your success, or your stories about the ways people mindlessly eat at www.MindlessEating.org.